HOW TO

Lower Blood Pressure Naturally

WITH ESSENTIAL OIL

WHAT HYPERTENSION IS,
CAUSES OF HIGH BLOOD PRESSURE
SYMPTOMS AND FAST REMEDIES

By Rebecca Park Totilo

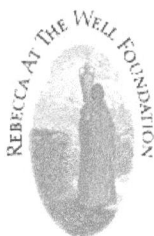

How to Lower Blood Pressure Naturally with Essential Oil

Printed in the United States of America.

Published by Rebecca at the Well Foundation, PO Box 60044, St. Petersburg, Florida 33784.

Disclaimer Notice: The information contained in this book is intended for educational purposes only and is not meant to substitute for medical care or prescribe treatment for any specific health condition. Please see a qualified health care provider for medical treatment. We assume no responsibility or liability for any person or group for any loss, damage or injury resulting from the use or misuse of any information in this book. No express or implied guarantee is given regarding the effects of using any of the products described herein.

ISBN 978-0-9898280-0-0

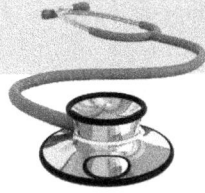

TABLE OF CONTENTS

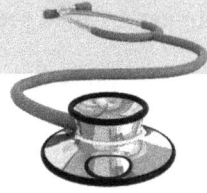

WHAT IS HIGH BLOOD PRESSURE?

Bump bump. Bump bump. Each time your heart beats, it is pumping blood into the arteries. Blood pressure is the force of the blood pushing against the walls of your arteries. Hypertension is another term used to describe high blood pressure.

Blood pressure readings are given in two numbers such as 120/80 mmHg. Your blood pressure is the highest when your heart beats, pumping the blood (in this example 120). This is called systolic pressure. When your heart is at rest, between beats, your blood pressure drops (in this example 80). This is called diastolic pressure. One or both of these numbers can be too high.

When your blood pressure is taken, a reading will use the systolic number first (the top number) and the diastolic number second (the bottom number).

Blood Pressure Reading:

- 119/79 or lower is normal blood pressure
- 140/90 or higher is high blood pressure
- Between 120 and 139 for the top number, or between 80 and 89 for the bottom number is called prehypertension

Prehypertension is an indication that you could end up with high blood pressure, unless steps are taken to prevent it. And, since high blood pressure has no symptoms, you will need to continually monitor it so that you do not end up with serious problems such as stroke, heart failure, heart attack and/or kidney failure. Individuals with prehypertension can also benefit from using essential oils to control their blood pressure along with healthy lifestyle habits.

Normal blood pressure is when your blood pressure is lower than 120/80 mmHg most of the time. High blood pressure is when your blood pressure is 140/90 mmHg or above most of the time. Prehypertension is when your blood pressure numbers are 120/80 or higher, but below 140/90. Depending on your health condition, your doctor may want to see your numbers lower, based on your current health condition.

WHAT CAUSES HIGH BLOOD PRESSURE?

There are several factors that can affect your blood pressure including:

- The amount of water and salt in your body
- The condition of your kidneys, nervous system, and blood vessels
- Your hormone levels

As people get older, it is possible to see an increase in blood pressure due to the vessels becoming stiffer with age. Other individuals who are at risk of high blood pressure include:

- African Americans
- Overweight and obese people
- Individuals who are often stressed or anxious
- Individuals who drink too much alcohol
- Individuals with a family history of high blood pressure
- Smokers
- Individuals with diabetes

- Individuals on high sodium diet

In some cases, high blood pressure is caused by another medical condition or medication. This is called secondary hypertension and may be caused by:

- Chronic kidney disease
- Disorders of the adrenal gland (such as Cushing syndrome or pheochromocytoma)
- Hyperparathyroidism
- Pregnancy or preeclampsia
- Medications (such as diet pills, birth control pills, cold medicines, migraine medications)
- Narrowed artery that supplies blood to the kidney (such as renal artery stenosis)

SYMPTOMS OF HIGH BLOOD PRESSURE

As stated earlier, most of the time people are unaware that they have high blood pressure because there are no visible symptoms. Usually, most people find out about their condition when they visit the doctor for another reason or have it checked elsewhere.

Undetected high blood pressure can result in damage to the heart or kidney problems. However, if you do suffer from severe headaches, nausea, vomiting, changes in vision, or nosebleeds, you may have a dangerous form of high blood pressure called malignant hypertension.

Other symptoms that may occur include: persistent morning headaches, dizziness, raised blood pressure (normal is about 120/80 systole/diastole), sweating, rapid pulse, shortness of breath, swollen ankles, or elevated cholesterol. You will want to see your doctor right away to be checked.

GETTING CHECKED FOR HIGH BLOOD PRESSURE

All adults should have their blood pressure checked annually if their blood pressure was less than 120/80 mmHg at their last reading. If you have high blood pressure, diabetes, kidney problems, or another health condition, you will want to have your high blood pressure checked more often. Your health care provider will measure your blood pressure several times before diagnosing you with high blood pressure. It is normal for your blood pressure to vary at different times a day. Readings performed at home with proper equipment will give you a more accurate reading of your current blood pressure than one taken at a grocery store, a fire station or doctor's office.

BLOOD PRESSURE MONITORING

You will need to purchase a good quality well-fitting home device to keep track of your blood pressure at home. A device can be purchased at a local pharmacy or online. Make sure it has one adjustable cuff for your arm and a digital readout. Practice with your health care provider to make sure you are taking your blood pressure properly to ensure you are getting accurate readings.

If you try taking your blood pressure throughout the day, you will notice that your pressure is usually higher while on the job, then drops when you are home. While sleeping, your blood pressure is usually the lowest. It is normal for your blood pressure to increase suddenly when you wake up. This is why people with high blood pressure are at risk for a heart attack or stroke in the early morning.

FOLLOW UP

You will want to monitor your blood pressure at home daily and keep a written record, along with any changes you make to your lifestyle, diet modifications and any essential oil regimens you incorporate into your daily routine. This is especially important to do once you have been diagnosed with high blood pressure by your doctor at a physical exam. Bring this information along with results to your next clinic visit. This will help the physician know what adjustments need to be made to your medications, if any have been prescribed.

Be sure to keep track of:

- Most recent blood pressure reading (note any increase in systolic and diastolic numbers)
- Time of day reading was performed
- Diet modifications, if any
- Physical exercises and/or changes in activity
- Essential oils used, how many drops, method of usage, times used

CHECKING BLOOD PRESSURE WHEN TRYING NEW BLENDS

When you begin using a new essential oil blend, you will want to check your blood pressure before and afterwards at varying intervals to measure its effect. To start out, check your blood pressure five minutes after applying oils, then one hour, then 8 hours, and so on. Record each test to see if you can see any measurable difference in your blood pressure. You may also want to try applying oils hourly and testing, then every 8 hours and then every 24 hours. Do not be discouraged if it takes some time to see results. Most people do, however, report immediate results after essential oils have been applied.

WHEN TO CALL THE DOCTOR

Do not hesitate to call your doctor if your blood pressure is abnormally high and well above your normal range. In addition, be sure to call your health care provider if you have any of these symptoms:

- Severe headache
- Irregular heartbeat or pulse
- Chest pain
- Sweating, nausea, or vomiting
- Shortness of breath
- Dizziness or lightheadedness
- Pain or tingling in the neck, jaw, shoulder, or arms
- Numbness or weakness in your body
- Fainting
- Trouble seeing
- Confusion
- Difficulty speaking
- Side effects caused by the medication you have been prescribed or your blood pressure

HOW TO TAKE AN ACCURATE BLOOD PRESSURE READING

Sit in a chair that offers back support with your legs uncrossed and your feet on the floor. Be sure your arm is supported so that your upper arm is at heart level. Wrap the blood pressure cuff around your bare upper arm (roll up your sleeve if necessary). The lower edge of the cuff should be approximately one inch above the bend of your elbow.

The cuff will inflate with air either by squeezing a bulb (manually) or pushing a button (electronically). You will feel tightness around the arm. Once the valve of the cuff opens slightly, the pressure will slowly fall. As the pressure falls, the reading for the systolic pressure begins when the first sound of the blood pulsing is heard. As the air continues to be let out, the point in which the sound stops is the diastolic pressure.

You may want to do the test two or three times to get a range of what your blood pressure is. Wait one minute between each reading. If the cuff is not inflated properly, you may get a false reading. You will want to check your blood pressure at the same time each day, such as in the morning and at night, to get an idea of what "normal" is for you.

GETTING ACCURATE RESULTS

Before taking your blood pressure, be sure to:

- Rest for at least five minutes before measuring your blood pressure.
- Wait until you are calm and collected. Do not take when you are under stress or just finished exercising.
- Wait thirty minutes after drinking a caffeinated drink or smoking tobacco.
- Compare your results with those of your health care provider to make sure your equipment is accurate.

TIP: In a hypertensive individual, small fluctuations in blood pressure is generally not harmful. However, prolonged moderate increases can be harmful, especially if they occur on a regular basis.

CONTROLLING YOUR HIGH BLOOD PRESSURE

In many cases, your health care provider may prescribe medications to help control your blood pressure. These medications, however, are not able to cure or fix the problem. Medications are prescribed to simply try to "control" your blood pressure. In more than 50% of patients taking medication, studies show that drugs are ineffective and cause numerous other complication.

There are other natural alternatives in which you can take an active role in regarding your health.

DIET, EXERCISE, AND OTHER LIFESTYLE CHANGES

- Limit the amount of sodium (salt) you eat to less than 1,500 mg per day.
- Limit how much alcohol you drink – 1 drink a day for women, 2 a day for men.
- Eat a heart-healthy diet, including potassium and fiber. Drink plenty of water.
- Stay at a healthy body weight. Get on a weight-loss program if necessary.
- Exercise regularly – at least 30 minutes a day of moderate aerobic exercise.
- Reduce stress by avoiding things that cause it. Try meditation or take a yoga class.
- Quit smoking.
- Increase your intake of magnesium. This acts as a smooth-muscle relaxant and as a natural calcium channel blocker for the heart, which helps lower blood pressure and dilate blood vessels.
- Use the recommended essential oils that are hypotensive two to three times a day.
- Consider doing an annual liver and colon cleanse for better circulation.

TREATMENT

After having a physical exam, your health care provider may look for signs of heart disease, damage to the eyes and other changes to the body. Tests may be performed for high cholesterol levels, heart disease such as an echocardiogram or electrocardiogram, and for kidney diseases such as urinalysis or an ultrasound of the kidneys. Since most patients that suffer from diabetes also have high blood pressure, it is possible they will want to check for diabetes as well.

If you have pre-hypertension, your health care provider may recommend lifestyle changes to try to normalize your blood pressure. Medicines are not normally recommended for pre-hypertension. This, however, is the ideal time to start using essential oils to help get your blood pressure in the normal range again.

If the results show you do suffer from high blood pressure, it will be critical to reduce your blood pressure so that you have a lower risk of complications to deal with down the road. If a doctor does prescribe medicine, oftentimes a single blood pressure medicine will not be enough to control your blood pressure and you will need to take two or more drugs. It is critical you take your medication as prescribed while using the essential oils. Wait until you see a noticeable change in your blood pressure on a regular basis and are able to return to the doctor to verify that you no longer need to take medicine. If you experience side effects from taking the drugs, you should go back to your health care provider and make them aware of this.

When blood pressure is not well controlled, you are at risk for:

- Bleeding from the aorta, the large blood vessel that supplies blood to the abdomen, pelvis, and legs
- Kidney disease
- Heart attack and heart failure
- Poor blood supply to the legs
- Problems with your vision
- Stroke

Even if you have not been diagnosed with high blood pressure, it is important to have your blood pressure checked during your yearly check-up, especially if someone in your family has or had high blood pressure.

HIGH BLOOD PRESSURE DURING PREGNANCY

If you are pregnant, high blood pressure can occur called gestational hypertension. This can cause problems for you and the baby if left unchecked. This can cause low birth weight or premature delivery of the baby. It is important to get prenatal care for the health of you and your baby. Treatments for high blood pressure during pregnancy need to be monitored, as well as changes in diet and prescribed medications.

According to the National Heart, Lung, and Blood Institute, some pregnant women with high blood pressure develop preeclampsia. This happens around the 20th week of pregnancy when there is a sudden increase in blood pressure. This can be life threatening for the mother and baby. This condition must be closely monitored to avoid complications, as the only way to "cure" it is to deliver the baby.

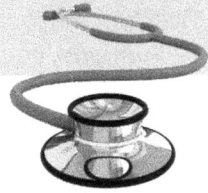

WHAT IS AN ESSENTIAL OIL?

Before examining how essential oils can help alleviate and lower blood pressure, let's first look at what an essential oil is and how it works.

Essential oils are a fragrant, vital fluid distilled from flowers, shrubs, leaves, trees, roots, and seeds. Because they are necessary for the life of the plant and play a vital role in the biological processes of the vegetation, these substances are called "essential." They carry the life-blood, intelligence, and vibrational energy that endow them with the healing power to sustain their own life—and help the people who use them.

TIP: Before using essential oils for any health condition, be sure to study each essential oils' profile to learn how each one works in general, as well as learn about their unique characteristics.

Since essential oils are derived from a natural plant source, you will notice that the oil does not leave an "oily" or greasy spot. Unlike fatty vegetable oils used for cooking (composed of molecules too large to penetrate at a cellular level), essential oils are a non-greasy liquid composed of tiny molecules that can permeate every cell and administer healing at the most fundamental level of our body. Their unique chemical makeup allows them to pass through the skin and the cell membranes where most needed. Whether diffused into the air or applied to the skin, they immediately are absorbed and go straight to action and are able to perform various functions.

Modern medicine has attempted to replicate the chemical constituents and healing capabilities of essential oils, but cannot. This is because man-made pharmaceuticals lack the intelligence and life-force found in the healing oils. Most synthetic prescriptions have several undesirable side effects—even some that are detrimental.

In general, essential oils have no serious side effects that are deadly. Many people have reported authentic healing when using them—though everyone may not experience the same results as family history, lifestyle, and diet plays a significant role in the body's healing process. Essential oils work together in harmony, making them inherently safe, unlike when multiple prescription drugs are taken, causing drug-interaction.

Some of the aromatic plants and their parts in which essential oils come from include trees, grasses, fruit, leaves, flowers, bark, needles, roots and seeds.

In addition, all essential oils have their own unique medicinal properties, characteristics and therapeutic benefits that will differ depending on the soil, climate, and altitude of the countries where the plants were grown.

Plant substances that have been extracted into essential oils are used in aromatherapy to promote well-being and good health. While the term aromatherapy can seem ambiguous, "scent" is only one aspect of aromatherapy, as you will discover many more dramatic benefits for healing the body, mind and spirit.

Special Note

It is important that you use only pure, unadulterated essential oils for therapeutic use.

In the aromatherapy industry, there is mass production of fragrances for multiple uses such as cosmetics, food and beverage flavoring, and home fragrances. For these uses there is less need that oils be "pure" and more need for consistency in its scent and it becomes likely oils may be introduced to synthetics and altered to meet standardization needs. Because of this, you will not want to purchase essential oils from department stores or big-chain health food stores, but instead obtain oils from a reputable company that provides quantifiable tests such as Gas Chromatography and Mass Spectroscopy that verify the oil's purity. Ask about these reports when purchasing your oils.

TIP: The FDA only requires an oil to contain 10% essential oil in order to be labeled, "100% Pure." Because of the absence of regulatory standards, some companies have added the terms "therapeutic grade" and "certified pure therapeutic grade" to their labels in hopes of gaining consumer confidence that their product has been developed with a higher standard of quality control and by labeling it as such represents their guarantee of being 100% pure. Please note though, all quality essential oils will not necessarily label their products as such, so it will be necessary for you to become educated in knowing how to determine which essential oils come from pure aromatic extracts and those that may contain fillers and non-aromatic compounds.

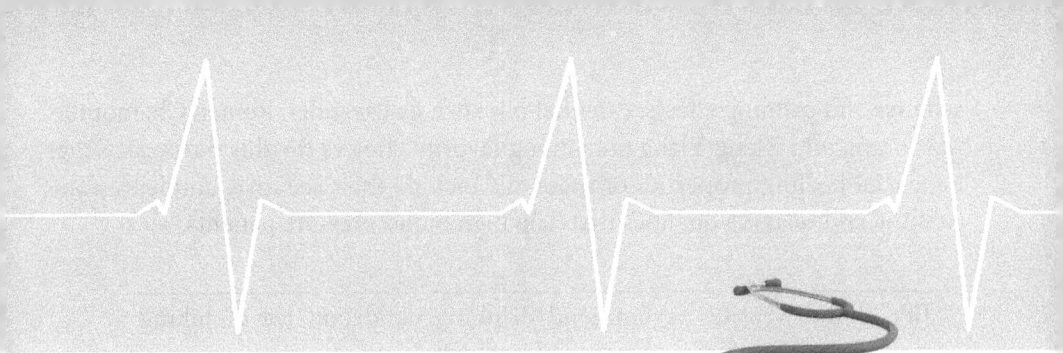

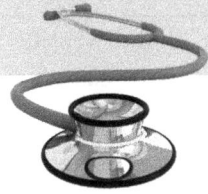

HOW ESSENTIAL OILS HELP
REDUCE
HIGH BLOOD
PRESSURE

Incorporating essential oils and natural remedies such as aromatherapy and relaxation techniques into your life can be very beneficial for a number of health conditions. To begin, aromatherapy helps support the treatment for high blood pressure by inducing relaxation and calming properties through aromatic baths and massages. Inhalation of certain essential oils is quite beneficial.

Many people with high blood pressure can benefit from certain essential oils that are hypotensive by nature. This unique chemical action within particular oils give them the ability to lower and regulate blood pressure. Along with an oil's sedative and calming effects, essential oils such as Lavender, Roman Chamomile, Marjoram, and Ylang Ylang are among favorite choices for this purpose. Other beneficial healing properties of these oils include their sedative, antidepressant, calming and relaxing qualities that help high blood pressure patients.

TIP: Some websites recommend drinking dandelion tea or taking garlic capsules to lower blood pressure.

Since untreated hypertension can lead to more serious health issues such as heart disease, it is important to combine your usage of essential oils with diet and lifestyle changes in order to achieve success with your natural remedy. In addition, you will want to address any stress or tension being experienced at home or work, as this can further exasperate the cause of high blood pressure. Many of these essential oils are effective for this purpose as well, and can offer immediate relief. For this reason, you will want to find several methods to incorporate them into your daily life.

Be sure to check with your doctor before using essential oils. It is important to make sure your health care provider is aware of your choice to use essential oils, so that any other medical conditions and/or prescription medications that may have contraindications can be monitored.

SPECIAL NOTE: Essential oils are not a "magic bullet." The suggestions of usage of essential oils in this book are for you to use as complementary care to the healthcare plan you already have in place. It may be necessary for you to make changes in a proper diet and other lifestyle modifications in order for all things to work together. High blood pressure is a very serious health concern and should be treated properly. If you do not achieve satisfactory results in normalizing your blood pressure, please seek professional medical help.

ESSENTIAL OIL PRECAUTIONS

If you have read any aromatherapy books or browsed any essential oil websites online, you will find most caution users to avoid certain essential oils with various health conditions, including high blood pressure. Many list essential oils such as Peppermint, Eucalyptus, Black Pepper, Pine, Rosemary, Hyssop, Sage and Thyme as contraindicated for people with high blood pressure. However, according to an article entitled, *Essential oils and hypertension - is there a problem?* author Robert Tisserand states that at closer examination of the research done in the 1940s, these oils actually reduce blood pressure. This "telephone game" of misinformation (simply repeating what another one says without any validity) resulted due to a French book published in 1964 by Jean Valnet. Tisserand says, "In other essential oils, the effects on vascular tone depend on whether they are ingested, rubbed on the skin, or inhaled. Ultimately, there is currently no compelling evidence that any essential oil is dangerous to use in hypertension." So, it simply could be a matter of which method of application is employed for these particular essential oils for high blood pressure patients.

For aromatherapy users seeing these same warnings plastered all over the Internet, they may still experience lingering doubts as to who they should believe when research is contradictory and seldom supported, or actual clinical experience is absent. AuraCacia.com website suggests, "With the absence of critical studies with scientific overview it is wise to err on the side of caution." For novice users, this may be the simplest way for determining which oils are safe – axe those "questionable" essential oils and place them on their *personal Do Not Use* list. Done. But, the problem is the elephant is still in the room and is now showing up in every aromatherapist's selfie. Those who would call themselves "Aromatherapists" should be the most qualified in the actual uses and potential toxicities of essential oils, as one would expect those in the medical and pharmaceutical industry to be when it comes to writing drug prescriptions. A closer examination as to which essential oils are genuinely safe is necessary.

The following essential oils that are typically listed as "do not use" with high blood pressure include:

- Camphor
- Hyssop
- Rosemary
- Sage
- Thyme

Several essential oil websites include Sage and Thyme on the "Do Not Use" list, however, Tisserand's article stated both Sage and Thyme were hypotensive in nature and in fact, lowered blood pressure. He supported his statement with the following data, "When 1 g/kg body weight of alcohol saturated with sage oil was given iv to dogs there was no increase in BP, and in some cases a slight fall occurred (Caujolle and Franck 1945a). Similarly, an aqueous-alcoholic extract of sage caused a moderate but prolonged hypotensive effect in cats when given iv (Todorov et al 1984)."

Thyme oil was also reported as having hypotensive action according to an abstract of a Russian paper (Kulieva 1980). Tisserand said that this was consistent "with the calcium channel blocking properties (and therefore hypotensive) because of its major constituents thymol and carvacrol (Magyar et al 2004)." In addition, "Intravenous carvacrol is hypotensive in rats (Aydin et al 2007), and topically applied thymol is hypotensive in rabbits (Futami 1984)."

Another questionable oil with regards to its use with high blood pressure is Rosemary. It's interesting to note that a major constituent of Rosemary is 1,8-cineole, which is hypotensive. Tisserand's article cited how Rosemary oil "caused a 25% fall in systolic pressure when administered iv to dogs in an emulsion at 26.3 mg/kg (Northover and Verghese 1962) and similarly, intravenous 1,8-cineole was dose-dependently hypotensive in rats at 0.3-10 mg/kg (Lahlou et al 2002)." So, while Rosemary, Sage or Thyme may not be your oil of choice when choosing essential oils to treat high blood pressure, these oils shouldn't be avoided like the plague either, as some would suggest.

Similar debates regarding Camphor and Hyssop continue to swirl as to whether they are hypotensive or hypertensive. Test results showed an initial drop in blood pressure in animal testing with Camphor and Hyssop, followed by a rise of blood pressure. Other factors may have played in, but for this reason, these two are not recommended to use with high blood pressure.

Other oils such as Peppermint, Eucalyptus and Black Pepper are also hypotensive by nature. In fact, Peppermint oil when topically applied reduced blood pressure for a short period of time due to its cooling menthol effect on local tissues (Futami 1984, Ragan et al 2004), and its calcium channel blocking makes hypertensive action unlikely (Hills and Aaronson 1991). Tisserand concluded in his article, "Dermal administration of essential oil constituents can cause reductions in BP due to local effects." While Black Pepper lowered blood pressure when injected iv into rats (Touvay et al 1995), it has been noted to raise blood pressure by inhalation.

In conclusion, Eucalyptus, Camphor, Pine, Thyme and Peppermint oils should be scratched from cautionary lists and are not contraindicated in hypertension according to Tisserand's paper. Hyssop and Sage oils are only a risk in convulsant oral doses, but at lower doses are hypotensive. Keep in mind that the reason for possible risk for some hypertensive patients with these particular essential oils may be due to certain dose/route combinations. Therefore, essential oils like Hyssop, Pennyroyal, Tansy, and Wormwood are listed below as "oils to avoid," even though these oils can be used safely, if one simply respects the dose given and the method of application used.

Since many seeking help to regulate their blood pressure may be new to essential oils, Camphor, Hyssop, and Rosemary oils remain on the Do Not Use With High Blood Pressure list below, even though there is no evidence that any essential oils have adverse effects on the control of blood pressure in humans.

The following precautions are divided into two groups: Topically and Inhalation. Use these lists to help you determine which essential oils to avoid based on your health condition.

ESSENTIAL OIL PRECAUTIONS FOR TOPICAL APPLICATIONS

Do Not Use With High Blood Pressure: Camphor, Hyssop, Rosemary

Do Not Use These Oils Anytime: Bitter Almond, Boldo, Buchu, Cade, Calamus, Brown Camphor, Costus, Elecampane, Mustard, Pennyroyal, Rue, Sassafras, Thuja, and Vanilla

Oils That May Be Mucous Membrane Irritants: Allspice, Cinnamon, Clove Bud, Oregano, Savory, Spearmint, and Thyme (not linalool)

Oils Not Recommended For Use in Bath: Basil, Benzoin, Bergamot, Black Pepper, Clove Bud, Cinnamon, Eucalyptus, Lemon, Litsea cubeba (May Chang), Marjoram, Nutmeg, Orange, Oregano, Peppermint, Pine, Rosemary, Sage, Spearmint, Tarragon, and Thyme

Oils Not Recommended For Children Under 5 Years: Basil, Camphor, Cedarwood (*Cedrus atlantica*), Eucalyptus, Fennel, Hyssop, Geranium, Jasmine, Marjoram, Nutmeg, Rose, Rosemary, Sage, and Tarragon

Oils To Avoid With Diabetes: Angelica Root

Oils To Avoid With Epilepsy: Camphor, Eucalyptus, Fennel, Hyssop, Rosemary, Sage, and Wormwood

Oils To Avoid When Using Homeopathic Remedies: Black Pepper, Camphor, Eucalyptus, Peppermint, Rosemary, and Spearmint

Oils To Avoid With Kidney Disease: Juniper Berry

Oils To Avoid With Low Blood Pressure: Clary Sage, Lavender, Marjoram, and Ylang Ylang

Oils Not Recommended For Long Term Use (more than 10 days in a row): Black Pepper, Fennel, Juniper Berry, Marjoram, and Tarragon

Oils To Avoid During Pregnancy: Anise Star, Aniseed, Basil, Bay Laurel, Birch, Bitter Almond, Camphor, Citronella, Cistus, Clary Sage, Clove Bud, Cedarwood, Cinnamon, Cumin, Cypress, Eucalyptus, Fennel, Frankincense, Hyssop, Indian Ginger, Jasmine, Juniper Berry, Marjoram, Mugwort, Myrrh, Nutmeg, Oregano, Pennyroyal, Rosemary, Sage, Tansy, Tarragon, Thyme, and Wintergreen

Oils Not Recommended For Sensitive Skin (or should be diluted): Aniseed, Basil, Bay Laurel, Bergamot, Black Pepper, Cajeput, Camphor, Citronella, Clove Bud, Fennel, Geranium, Ginger, Grapefruit, Lemon, Lemongrass, Lime, Mandarin, Orange, Oregano, Rosemary, Peppermint, Petitgrain, Pine, Pimento Leaf, Savory, Spearmint, Spruce, Thyme, Oregano, and Wintergreen

Oils That May Be Photo-Toxic or Cause Sun Sensitivity: Angelica Root, Bergamot, Cumin, Grapefruit, Lemon, Lime, Mandarin, Melissa, Opoponax, Orange, and Verbena

Oils That May Be Potentially Toxic: Ajowan, Bitter Almond, Inula, Khella, Mugwort (Wormwood), Pennyroyal, and Sassafras

Oils Considered Very Toxic: Arnica, Boldo, Buchu, Calamus, Cascarilla, Chervil, Camphor (brown), Deer Tongue, Horseradish, Jaborandi, Mustard, Narcissus, and Rue

Oils To Avoid With History of Estrogen-Dependent Cancer: Aniseed, Basil, Clary Sage, Cypress, Fennel, Geranium, Myrrh, Pine (prostate cancer), Sage, Tarragon, and Vitex

Oils To Avoid Long Term Use with Estrogen-Dependent Cancer: Roman Chamomile

Oils That May Increase Narcotic Effect of Alcohol: Clary Sage

ESSENTIAL OILS PRECAUTIONS FOR INHALATION

The following essential oils presented a slight risk of an increase of blood pressure temporary when administered through intense inhalation. This group mainly consists of oils high in carvone or limonene.

Oils To Avoid With High Blood Pressure: Grapefruit, Lemon, Caraway, Black Pepper, Fennel, Tarragon

SUPPORTING RESEARCH

The following information and links are just a sampling of research being conducted on the effects of essential oils. This is certainly good news for many who are seeking answers to this national health epidemic.

- Researchers in Korea found that subjects that wore special necklaces scented with an essential oil blend of Lavender, Ylang Ylang, Marjoram and Neroli had reduced blood pressure levels and lower salivary cortisol levels (http://www.ncbi.nlm.nih.gov/pmc/articles/PMC3521421/pdf/ECAM2012-984203.pdf).
- In a study conducted in Thailand, Lavender oil caused significant decreases of blood pressure and heart rate (http://www.ncbi.nlm.nih.gov/pubmed/22612017).
- In the United Kingdom, Aromatherapist Jolanta Basnyet conducted a study to reveal the connection between high blood pressure and essential oil treatments through massage. Significant improvement resulted (70%) for lowering blood pressure with the use of essential oils than those who did not. (http://www.positivehealth.com/article/aromatherapy/the-effect-of-aromatherapy-treatment-on-raised-arterial-blood-pressure)
- A journal was written on the Effects of Aromatherapy on the Anxiety, Vital Signs, and Sleep Quality of Percutaneous Coronary Intervention Patients in Intensive Care Units by Mi-Yeon Cho, Eun Sil Min, Myung-Haeng Hur, and Myeong Soo Lee. This study in Korea was designed to assess the effect of a Lavender, Roman Chamomile, and Neroli oil aromatherapy blend on anxiety, sleep, and blood pressure in coronary artery disease patients with ischemic heart diseases after a stent insertion during coronary angiography who were admitted to the ICU. https://www.scienceopen.com/document/vid/0f9192b0-d07f-452e-9ff7-89eba6ee7a27

- Argan (Argania spinosa) oil lowers blood pressure and improves endothelial dysfunction in spontaneously hypertensive rats; Berrougui H, Alvarez de Sotomayor M, Perez-Guerrero C, Ettaib A, Hmamouchi M, Marhuenda E, Herrera MD. http://www.ncbi.nlm.nih.gov/pubmed/15613254
- Psychiatry Research scientifically confirms the benefit of Lavender and Rosemary essential oils in reducing stress and related health problems. Smelling Lavender and Rosemary increases free radical scavenging activity and decreases cortisol level in saliva; Atsumi T, Tonosaki K. Department of Oral Physiology, Meikai University, School of Dentistry, 1-1, Keyaki-dai, Sakado-shi, Saitama 350-0283, Japan. http://www.psy-journal.com
- After 10 minutes of inhaling 14.2 μg of vaporized cedrol (a sesquiterpene alcohol found in the essential oil of conifers such as Cypress and Juniper Berry, those in the genera Cupressus and Juniperus.), both systolic and diastolic pressures were reduced in healthy male and female Japanese volunteers, due to a reduction in sympathetic and an increase in parasympathetic activity; Dayawansa S, Umeno K, Takakura H et al 2003 Autonomic responses during inhalation of natural fragrance of cedrol in humans. Autonomic Neuroscience 108:79-86

Other documented uses for the essential oils mentioned in this book include: Aneurysm, angina, arterial vasodilator, arteriosclerosis, arthritis, high blood pressure (hypertension), to stop bleeding, blood vessels, shortness of breath, cardiovascular system, chelation (plaque and metals), circulation, high cholesterol, dizziness, edema, drooping eye lids, headaches, heart tonic, joint stiffness/pain, large valve, palpitations (rapid and forceful contraction of the heart), hemorrhoids, hormonal system, kidneys, inflammation of kidney (nephritis), heart failure/ attack, lungs, pulmonary conditions, lymphatic system decongestant, memory, mental fatigue, migraine headaches, bruised muscles, phlebitis, skin elasticity, Raynaud's Disease, sciatica, shock, skin, stress, stroke (thrombotic), tachycardia (rapid heartbeat), toxemia, varicose veins, spider veins, and vascular system.

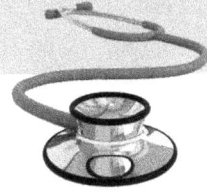

ESSENTIAL OILS RECOMMENDED FOR
HIGH BLOOD PRESSURE

The following is a list of essential oils that have historically been used to help regulate high blood pressure. All the essential oils mentioned here can easily be incorporated into daily life through inhalation, topical application and massage.

There are several oils to choose from; however, those that are immediate favorites among essential oil enthusiasts include Lavender (Lavandula angustifolia) because of its high content of esters and alcohols, chemically speaking. Its sweet, floral aroma is very calming and works as a general tonic on the nervous system. In addition to this, Lavender's soothing effect on the body as well as emotions makes it a favorite in the treatment of nervous disorders.

A second favorite is Sweet Marjoram (Origanum marjorana), which is high in monoterpenols and serves as a balancing tonic that is calming to the mind. It is great for chronic lethargy and nervous exhaustion. Sweet Marjoram's warm, spicy scent is quite relaxing and soothing.

Another essential oil that doesn't get quite as much fanfare is Cypress (Cupresus sepmervirens), which strengthens the vascular system and increases circulation while at the same time supports the detoxification of the lymphatic system. Quite beneficial indeed!

Helichrysum (Helichrysum italicum) is a powerhouse all by itself as a natural anti-inflammatory; it improves circulation and cleanses the blood. Finally, Ylang Ylang (Cananga odorata) which is high in sesquiterpenes, offers a calming and supportive effect to the nervous system while easing stress and tension that leads to high blood pressure. Like several of the previous essential oils mentioned, Ylang Ylang is high in alcohols and esters, which makes it rich in qualities such as promoting sleep and soothing agitation. Its sweet floral scent is quite intense, though, so you will not want to add too much of this oil to your blend. Kurt Schnaublet, PhD, in his book "Advanced Aromatherapy," states that even in the minutest amounts, Ylang Ylang has a noticeable and instantaneous effect on heart palpitations. Dr. James Howenstein, MD, recommends rubbing a single drop of Ylang Ylang oil between the fingertips and inhaling for one minute for hypertension. This can be repeated as needed.

There are many, many more essential oils to choose from. It is important, however, to check with your doctor before using essential oils. There are some medical conditions, such as prescription medications and pregnancy that contraindicate the use of some essential oils.

BAY LAUREL (Laurus nobilis) includes chemical constituents Cineole and Linalool and has antiseptic, antibiotic, analgesic, anti-neuralgic, astringent, insecticidal and sedative properties. Bay is used in the treatment of rheumatism, muscular pain, circulation problems, colds, flu, dental infections and skin infections. Bay's high eugenol content may irritate the skin and mucus membranes, so dilution is necessary. Avoid use during pregnancy. **Note:** Top

BERGAMOT (Citrus bergamia) helps to release pent up emotions and accumulated stress. It is commonly used in many skin care creams and lotions because of its refreshing citrus nature. It is ideal for helping to calm inflamed skin and is an ingredient in some creams for eczema and psoriasis. Bergamot's chemical makeup has antiseptic properties, which help ward off infection and aid recovery. It is a favorite oil of aromatherapists in treating depression. Bergamot is also effective as an antispasmodic and helps to reduce leg cramps and is used for restless leg syndrome. It is also suitable for coughs and works as a digestive aid. The therapeutic properties of Bergamot include analgesic, antidepressant, antiseptic, antibiotic, anti-spasmodic, stomachic, calmative, cicatrisant, deodorant, digestive, febrifuge, vermifuge and vulnerary. Bergamot essential oil has phototoxic properties; therefore exposure to the sun must be avoided after use. It may also interfere with the activity of certain prescription drugs. Note: Top

BLUE TANSY (Tanacetum annuum) has a surprisingly sweet scent making it ideal for applications in skin care products and skin therapies. Blue Tansy contains the active azulene, best known for its skin care properties and as an anti-inflammatory agent. It has been credited by aromatherapists as being antihistamine and antispasmodic. Blue Tansy is also excellent for reducing the effects of allergic reactions, asthma, and other skin allergies. This oil induces relaxation, reduces nervous tension and stress, and has hormone-like actions stimulating the thymus gland. Blue Tansy reduces fever, treats colds and other respiratory infections by boosting the immune system. It supports the balance of white blood cell production, nourishes the spleen, and may be helpful for leukemia. This oil is fabulous for the treatment of sprains, rheumatism, arthritis, and sciatica. It helps to stabilize blood sugar, eliminates bruises, itching, rashes, cysts, and reduces blood pressure. Its therapeutic properties include anthelmintic, vermifuge, carminative, digestive, anti-inflammatory, analgesic, antispasmodic, anti-allergic, antihistamine, febrifuge, diaphoretic, stimulant, tonic, antipruritic, emmenagogue, and hypotensive. Special attention should be given to its blue color as it may change cream or lotion colors. Blue Tansy essential oil is generally non-irritating and non-toxic. Avoid use during pregnancy. Note: Middle

CASSIA (Cinnamomum Cassia) has antiseptic properties that are known to kill various types of bacteria and fungi. Cassia has been used as a tonic, carminative and stimulant for treating nausea, flatulence and diarrhea. Chinese and Japanese scientists have found that Cassia's sedative effect lowers high blood pressure. The therapeutic properties of Cassia are carminative, anti-diarrhea, antimicrobial and anti-emetic. It is a dermal irritant, dermal sensitizer and a mucus membrane irritant. Avoid use during pregnancy. **Note:** Middle

CISTUS LABDANUM (Cistus Ladaniferus) contains antimicrobial, antiseptic, astringent and expectorant properties and acts as a fixative in perfumes as it is widely used in the perfumery industry. It is considered useful in skin care preparations especially for mature skin and wrinkles. Labdanum is known to heal wounds quickly. The Rock Rose's properties include being antiseptic, anti-infectious, anti-inflammatory, anti-tussive, astringent, cicatrisant, mucolytic, and a tonic for the nervous system. This oil is strongly highlighted in medical research at this time with studies at animal trial level into vasodilators with hypotensive patients and entry inhibitors in HIV. Uses for Cistus Labdanum include treating symptoms and effects of stress, infection, high blood pressure and anxiety. This oil is generally non-toxic and non-sensitizing. Avoid use during pregnancy. **Note:** Base

CLARY SAGE (Salvia sclarea) can be used as a deodorant, antidepressant, and a sedative. Its analgesic and antispasmodic actions can decrease heart rate (Buckle, 1997) and is considered mildly hypotensive (Rovesti and Gattefosse, 1973). It is effective in combating oily hair and is a superior oil for acne, wrinkles and fine lines. Women experiencing hormonal changes and menopause symptoms such as hot flashes find this oil quite beneficial. Clary Sage's properties are antidepressant, anticonvulsive, antispasmodic, antiseptic, aphrodisiac, astringent, bactericidal, carminative, deodorant, digestive, emmenagogue, euphoric, hypotensive, nervine, sedative, stomachic, uterine and nerve tonic. Clary Sage oil is non-toxic and non-sensitizing. Do not use during pregnancy or if you are at risk for breast cancer as it may have an estrogen-like effect on the body. **Note:** Top-Middle

CLOVE BUD (Syzgium aromaticum) has a spicy rich scent and is an effective agent for minor aches and pains, particularly dental pain because of its numerous effects on the oral tissues. Clove Bud can be used for acne, cuts and bruises, preventing infections and as a pain reliever. It helps with toothaches, mouth sores, rheumatism and arthritis. For the digestive system, it helps to prevent vomiting, diarrhea, flatulence, spasms and parasites, as well as bad breath. Clove oil is valuable for relieving respiratory problems, like bronchitis, asthma and tuberculosis. Its disinfecting feature makes it useful with infectious diseases. Clove oil's therapeutic properties are analgesic, antiseptic, antispasmodic, anti-neuralgic, carminative, anti-infectious, disinfectant, insecticide, tonic, stomachic, uterine, and stimulating. This oil may cause sensitization in some individuals and should be used in dilution. Avoid use during pregnancy. **Note:** Middle

CYPRESS (Cupressus sempervirens) is used to prevent excessive perspiration, particularly in the feet. It is good for hemorrhoids and oily skin, and acts as an astringent in skin care applications. It is extremely gentle and suitable for all skin types. This oil calms and soothes anger while having a positive effect on one's mood. It is suitable for various female problems and is good for coughs and bronchitis. Cypress assists with varicose veins and bodily fluids by improving circulation. Its properties include antibacterial, anti-infectious, anti-inflammatory, anti-rheumatic, antiseptic, antispasmodic, astringent, decongestant, diuretic, and vein tonic. Avoid use during pregnancy. Avoid long-term use with high-blood pressure. **Note**: Middle-Base

CYPRESS, BLUE (Callitris intratropicai) is popular for its moisturizing and soothing skin care properties. This oil is considered similar to German Chamomile due to its soothing and relaxing properties for the nerves without having sedative properties. The therapeutic properties of Cypress are astringent, antiseptic, antispasmodic, deodorant, diuretic, homeostatic, hepatic, styptic, sudorific, vasoconstrictor, respiratory tonic and sedative. It is considered non-toxic and non-irritant. Blue Cypress is regarded as very gentle and suitable for all skin types. Avoid use during pregnancy. **Note**: Middle-Base

FRANKINCENSE (Boswellia carterii) is highly prized in the aromatherapy industry. It is frequently used in skin care products' as it is considered a valuable ingredient having remarkable anti-aging, rejuvenating and healing properties. Frankincense is known to calm the mind and end mental chatter. It also helps to ease worry and agitation. The therapeutic properties of Frankincense oil are antiseptic, astringent, carminative, cicatrisant, cytophylactic, digestive, diuretic, emmenagogue, expectorant, sedative, tonic, uterine, and vulnerary. Frankincense is non-toxic, non-irritant and non-sensitizing. Avoid use during pregnancy. **Note**: Base

GARLIC (Allium sativum) has antibacterial, antiseptic and anti-hypertensive properties that can be used to prevent infections as well as treat colds, bronchitis and flu symptoms. It is also a powerful detoxifier and rejuvenates the body. Garlic is recognized as a preventative of high blood pressure and heart disease when taken internally. It is extremely effective at reducing high cholesterol levels. Garlic's antiseptic, bactericidal and detoxifying properties make it a valuable essential oil in treating acne. Garlic has been used for thousands of years to prevent infestation with intestinal worms, both in people and in animals, and is one of the best treatments for gastro-intestinal infections. As an antibiotic, Garlic does not kill off the beneficial flora of the intestine as synthetic antibiotics do and is an effective treatment for cystitis. This oil must be properly diluted. Avoid use during pregnancy. **Note**: Top

GERANIUM (Pelargonium graveolens) is used as an astringent, haemostatic, diuretic, antiseptic, antispasmodic and anti-infectious agent. This oil works wonders for wrinkles and is also indicated for disturbed and sensitive skin, as well as broken capillaries. It works well in reducing edema and fluid retention, promoting circulation and has a stimulating effect on the lymphatic system.

Geranium works well as a decent overall skin cleanser and makes a fabulous oil for mature and troubled skin, bringing a radiant glow to your complexion. Geranium is well tolerated by most individuals, but since it helps in balancing the hormonal system, care must be taken during pregnancy. Avoid use during the first and second trimester of pregnancy. Do not use if you have a history of estrogen-dependent cancer or are hypoglycemic. **Note:** Middle

GINGER (Zingiber officinale) is excellent for colds and flu, nausea (including motion sickness and morning sickness), rheumatism, coughs and circulation issues. It has warming properties that help to relieve muscular cramps, spasms, aches and eases stiffness in joints. Ginger's healing properties include analgesic, anti-inflammatory, antiseptic, antispasmodic, carminative, tonic, diaphoretic, expectorant, and antiemetic. It may irritate sensitive skin. Avoid use during pregnancy. **Note:** Base

GOLDENROD (Solidago virgaurea) is known to support the circulatory system, urinary tract, and liver function. It has relaxing and calming effects with anti-inflammatory, anti-hypertensive, diuretic, and liver tonic properties. Goldenrod is helpful for the cardiovascular system, bladder infection, congestive cough, diphtheria, diuretic, dyspepsia, fibrillation, heart tonic (stimulant), hypertension, hepatitis, impotence, influenza, fatty liver, liver congestion, nervousness, neuropathy, respiratory mucus, sleep disorders, tachycardia, tonsillitis, and pharyngitis. Goldenrod could possibly cause skin sensitivity. Avoid use during pregnancy. **Note:** Middle

HELICHRYSUM (Helichrysum italicum) is an effective oil for acne, bruises, boils, burns, cuts, dermatitis, eczema, irritated skin and wounds. It supports the body through post-viral fatigue and convalescence, and can also be used to repair skin damaged by psoriasis, eczema or ulceration. Helichrysum's therapeutic properties include anti-inflammatory, antibacterial, analgesic, antiseptic, antispasmodic, antifungal, antiviral, antimicrobial, and as a tonic for the nervous system. This oil is non-toxic, non-irritating and non-sensitizing. Please check with your healthcare provider before use during pregnancy. **Note:** Base

HO WOOD (Cinnamomum camphora) has antidepressant, antimicrobial, antiseptic, aphrodisiac, analgesic, anti-infectious, anti-inflammatory, antispasmodic, sedative, immune support, tonic and bactericidal properties. It also plays a role as a cellular stimulant, cephalic, and tissue regenerator. Ho Wood has become popular as a replacement for Rosewood because of similar chemical qualities. It may cause irritation to the skin. Avoid use during pregnancy. **Note:** Middle

JASMINE (Jasminum grandiflorum) is well respected for its aphrodisiac properties and is a sensual, soothing, calming oil that promotes love and peace. It is necessary to note that all absolutes are highly concentrated by nature. The complexity of the fragrance, particularly the rare and exotic notes, is well regarded as an antidepressant, antiseptic, cicatrisant, expectorant, galactagogue, parturient, sedative, uterine and antispasmodic. Avoid use during the first and second trimester of pregnancy. **Note:** Base

LAVANDIN (Lavandula intermedia var Abrialis) properties include analgesic, anti-convulsive, antidepressant, anti-phlogistic, anti-rheumatic, antiseptic, antispasmodic, antiviral, bactericidal, carminative, cholagogue, cicatrisant, cordial, cytophylactic, decongestant, deodorant, and diuretic. It is considered one of the most useful and versatile essential oils; it eases sore muscles and joints, relieves muscle stiffness, clears the lungs and sinuses from phlegm, heals wounds and clears dermatitis. Lavandin is advantageous for burns and healing of the skin. Its antiseptic and analgesic properties aid with easing pain and preventing infection. Lavandin cytophylactic properties promote rapid healing and help reduce scarring. Its calming scent reduces anxiety and promotes sleep. This oil is non-toxic, non-irritating and non-sensitizing. **Note:** Middle

LAVENDER (Lavandula angustifolia) is most commonly used for burns and the healing of skin. It has antiseptic and analgesic properties that eases the pain of a burn and prevents infection. Lavender also has cytophylactic properties that promote rapid healing and reduce scarring. Lavender does an excellent job at balancing oil production in the skin as well as clearing blemishes and evening skin tone, and even helps to hydrate dry skin. Lavender is indicated for all skin types and can be used at any step in your skin care regimen. Lavender is beneficial for colds, flu, asthma, high blood pressure, and migraines. It is also excellent for helping with insomnia. The therapeutic properties of Lavender oil are antiseptic, analgesic, anti-convulsant, antidepressant, anti-rheumatic, antispasmodic, anti-inflammatory, antiviral, bactericide, carminative, cholagogue, cicatrisant, cordial, cytophylactic, decongestant, deodorant, diuretic, emmenagogue, hypotensive, nervine, rubefacient, sedative, sudorific and vulnerary. Lavender is non-toxic, non-irritating and non-sensitizing. Do not use during the first trimester of pregnancy. **Note:** Middle

LEMON (Citrus Limon) is recognized as a cleanser and antiseptic with refreshing and cooling properties. For the skin and hair, Lemon is used for its cleansing effect, as well as for treating cuts and boils. This oil's fresh scent is treasured for improving concentration, reducing acidity in the body while assisting with digestion and eliminating cellulite, rheumatism, arthritis and gout. It is beneficial for the circulatory system and aids with blood flow, reduces blood pressure and helps with nosebleeds. Lemon oil can be used to help reduce a fever, relieve throat infections and bronchitis, and heal cold sores, herpes and insect bites. Lemon's therapeutic properties are anti-anemic, antimicrobial, anti-rheumatic, anti-sclerotic, antiseptic, bactericidal, carminative, cicatrisant, depurative, diaphoretic, diuretic, febrifuge, haemostatic, hypotensive, insecticidal, rubefacient, tonic and vermifuge. Lemon is non-toxic but may cause skin irritation for some. It is also phototoxic and should be avoided prior to exposure to direct sunlight. **Note**: Top

MARJORAM (Origanum marjorana) is known for helping combat stress and anxiety. Marjoram's chemical constituents of aldehydes, in the form of citral and geranyl acetate, aid in lowering the blood pressure (Tiran, 1996). It is a comforting oil that can be massaged into the abdomen during menstruation, or added to a warm compress to ease discomfort. It is useful for treating tired aching muscles or in a sports massage. Marjoram's pain relieving properties are useful for rheumatic pains, sprains, and spasms, as well as swollen joints and achy muscles. It can be added to a warm or hot bath at the first sign of a cold. This oil is helpful for asthma and other respiratory complaints and has a calming effect on emotions, especially for hyperactive people. It soothes the digestive system and helps with indigestion, constipation and flatulence. Marjoram is superb as a relaxant and is useful for headaches, migraines and insomnia. Marjoram is relaxing and quiets the mind and obsessive over-thinking. Marjoram's therapeutic properties are analgesic, antispasmodic, anaphrodisiac, antiseptic, antiviral, bactericidal, carminative, cephalic, cordial, diaphoretic, digestive, diuretic, emmenagogue, expectorant, fungicidal, hypotensive, laxative, nervine, sedative, stomachic, vasodilator and vulnerary. It can also be used in masculine, oriental, and herbal-spicy perfumes and colognes. Marjoram is generally non-toxic, non-irritating and non-sensitizing. Use with caution if you have low blood pressure. Avoid use during pregnancy. **Note**: Middle

MELISSA (Melissa officinalis) also commonly called Lemon Balm, is well known for its antidepressant and uplifting properties. Its healing properties include antidepressant, anti-inflammatory, antiviral, antispasmodic, bactericidal, carminative, cordial, diaphoretic, emmenagogue, nervine, sedative, stomachic, sudorific, and tonic. Melissa has strong sedative qualities and treats emotional trauma and shock. It is considered non-sensitizing and non-toxic. Please check with your healthcare provider before use during pregnancy. **Note**: Middle-Top

NEROLI (Citrus aurantium) increases circulation and stimulates new cell growth. It prevents scarring and stretch marks, and is useful in treating skin conditions linked to emotional stress. Any type of skin can benefit from this oil, although it is particularly nourishing for dry, irritated or sensitive skin. Neroli regulates oiliness, minimizes enlarged pores, and helps clear acne and blemished skin, especially if the skin lacks moisture. With regular treatment, it can reduce the appearance of fragile or broken capillaries and varicose veins. Neroli is useful for dry, sensitive and mature skin as it helps improves elasticity. It is also known to help relieve muscle spasms and heart palpitations. It provides comfort and strength emotionally and helps to release repressed emotions. Neroli's therapeutic properties are antidepressant, antiseptic, anti-infectious, antispasmodic, aphrodisiac, bactericidal, carminative, cicatrisant, cytophylactic, cordial, deodorant, digestive, sedative and tonic. This oil is non-toxic and non-sensitizing. Avoid use during pregnancy. **Note**: Middle-Top

OREGANO (Origanum vulgare) is considered nature's cure-all due to its high carvacrol and thymol content. This oil's potent properties include antiviral, antifungal, antibacterial and anti-parasitic. In topical applications, it can be used to treat itches, skin infections, cuts and wounds. Oregano's anti-inflammatory properties make it effective against swelling and pain caused by rheumatism. It can be used as a fragrance component in soaps, colognes and perfumes, especially men's fragrances. Oregano is both a dermal irritant and a mucous membrane irritant. Avoid use during pregnancy. **Note**: Top

PETITGRAIN (Citrus aurantium) is believed to have uplifting properties and is used for calming anger and stress. It is commonly used in the skin care industry for acne, oily skin, and as a deodorizing agent. Petitgrain is valued for its ability to reduce pain and spasms in the lower intestines. Its calming qualities make it a favorite for insomnia. This oil's properties include antidepressant, antiseptic, antispasmodic, deodorant, immuno-support and stimulant, tonic and sedative for the nervous system. Petitgrain is generally considered non-toxic, non-irritant, and non-sensitizing. **Note**: Top

ROMAN CHAMOMILE (Anthemis nobilis) helps relieve nervous stress of any kind, while easing frustration, resentment and depression. It is good for most skin types, acne, allergies, boils, burns, eczema, inflamed skin conditions, wounds, menstrual pain, premenstrual syndrome, headache, insomnia, restless leg syndrome, and nervous tension. The therapeutic properties of Roman Chamomile oil are analgesic, antispasmodic, antiseptic, antibiotic, anti-inflammatory, anti-infectious, antidepressant, antineuralgic, antiphlogistic, antiseptic, antispasmodic, bactericidal, carminative, cholagogue, cicatrisant, emmenagogue, febrifuge, hepatic, sedative, nervine, digestive, tonic, sudorific, stomachic, vermifuge and vulnerary. It is non-toxic and non-irritant. This oil should not be used by anyone who is allergic to ragweed. Avoid use during the first and second trimester of pregnancy. **Note**: Middle

ROSE has a soothing quality for inflammation and constricting action on capillaries. Rose oil is used in the treatment for depression, grief, anger and other unpleasant emotions. It supports the heart and digestive systems and is considered one of the most incredible remedy's for female problems such as balancing hormones during menopause. The therapeutic properties of Rose are antidepressant, antiphlogistic, antiseptic, antispasmodic, antiviral, aphrodisiac, astringent, bactericidal, choleretic, cicatrisant, depurative, emmenagogue, haemostatic, hepatic, laxative, nervous system sedative, stomachic and a tonic for the heart, liver, stomach and uterus. Avoid use during the first trimester of pregnancy. **Note**: Base

SPIKENARD (Nardostachys jatamansi) is used by aromatherapists for rashes, wrinkles, cuts, insomnia, migraines, and wounds. It brings peaceful tranquility. This oil's therapeutic properties are anti-inflammatory, antifungal, antispasmodic, sedative and tonic. Spikenard should be avoided during pregnancy. **Note**: Base

TURMERIC (Curcuma longa) is viewed as a strong relaxant and balancer. It has historical applications as an antiseptic aid for skin care used in treating acne and facial hair in women. It is an analgesic for painful joint conditions such as rheumatism. This oil makes a wonderful digestive aid and helps to reduce excess fluid. Its therapeutic properties include analgesic, anti-inflammatory, carminative, tonic, and diuretic. Turmeric has potential irritating and toxic effects when used in large concentrations. Avoid use during pregnancy. **Note**: Base

VALERIAN (Valeriana officinalis) is used to combat insomnia, nervousness, restlessness, tension, agitation, panic attacks, and headaches as the result of nervous tension. It has also been used on muscle spasms, heart palpitations, cardiovascular spasms and neuralgia. Valerian is a suitable replacement for catnip based on similar chemical components and is gaining popularity as a natural alternative to commercially available sedatives. The therapeutic properties of Valerian are antispasmodic, bactericidal, carminative, diuretic, hypnotic, hypotensive, regulator, sedative, and stomachic. It has possible skin sensitizing properties, though it is non-toxic and non-irritating at low doses. Avoid use during pregnancy and with children. **Note**: Base

YARROW (Achillea millefolium) is credited with having an energy similar to that of the earth. It is a balancing, uplifting oil with practical applications on gynecological issues, wounds and open sores. This oil is used in cosmetics for dry skin care and is an exceptional oil for reducing swelling, muscle spasms, digestive issues, indigestion, irritable bowel syndrome, and flatulence. It is also beneficial as an anti-inflammatory for muscle and joint conditions. The therapeutic properties of Yarrow are analgesic, anti-allergenic, antidepressant, anti-inflammatory, antiseptic, antiviral, cicatrisant, decongestant, digestive aid and diuretic. Yarrow has no known toxicity and is non-irritant in low concentration. **Note:** Middle

YLANG YLANG (Cananga odorata) assists with problems such as high blood pressure due to its content of alcohols and cadinene, which is hypotensive (Tiran 1996), rapid breathing and heartbeat, nervous conditions, as well as impotence and frigidity. Ylang Ylang is renowned as a treatment for arterial hypertension and tachycardia (Rose, 1994). This oil is best suited for use in the perfumery and skin care industries due to it having a balancing effect on sebum and is useful for both oily and dry skin types. The therapeutic properties of Ylang Ylang are antidepressant, antiseborrheic, antiseptic, aphrodisiac, hypotensive, nervine and sedative. Ylang Ylang may cause sensitivity in some people and excessive use of it may lead to headaches and nausea. This oil is not recommended if you have low blood pressure. **Note:** Base

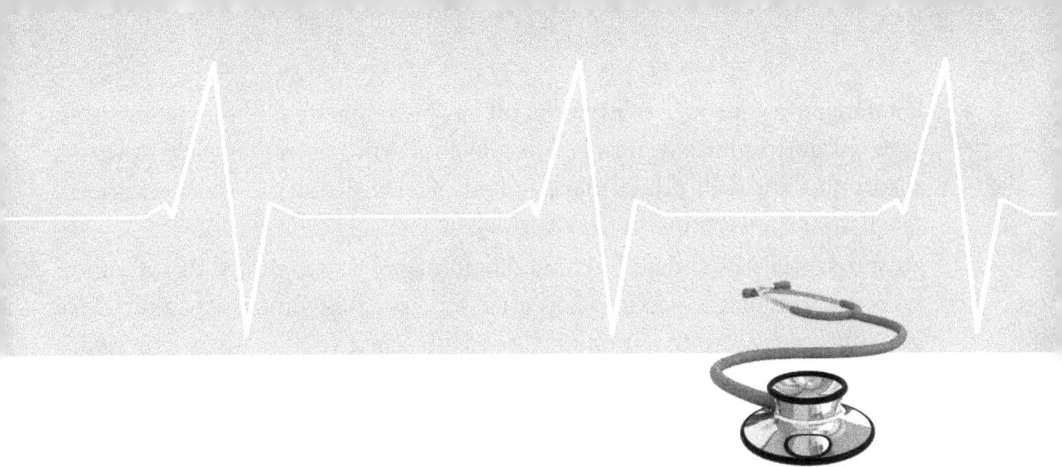

ESSENTIAL
OIL SAFETY

In general, essential oils are safe to use for aromatherapy and therapeutic purposes. Nevertheless, safety must be exercised due to their potency and high concentration. Please read and follow these guidelines to obtain the maximum effectiveness and benefits.

- Avoid sunbathing, tanning booths, or saunas immediately after using essential oils.
- Be careful to avoid getting essential oils in the eyes. If you do splash a drop or two of essential oil in the eyes, use a small amount of olive oil (or another carrier oil) to dilute the essential oil and absorb with a washcloth. If serious, seek medical attention immediately.
- Take extra precaution when using oils with children. Never use undiluted essential oils on babies and always store your essential oils out of the reach of children.
- Never take essential oils internally, unless advised by your medical practitioner or another qualified health professional.

- If a dangerous quantity of essential oil has been ingested, immediately drink olive oil and induce vomiting. The olive oil will help in slowing down its absorption and will dilute the essential oil. Do not drink water—this will speed up the absorption of the essential oil.

- Most essential oils should be diluted before applying topically. Pay attention to safety guidelines—certain essential oils, such as Cinnamon and Clove Bud, may cause skin irritation for those with sensitive skin. If you experience slight redness or itchiness, put olive oil (or any carrier oil) on the affected area and cover with a soft cloth. The olive oil acts as an absorbent fat and binds to the oil diluting its strength and allowing it to be immediately removed. Aloe Vera gel also works well as an alternative to olive oil. Never use water to dilute essential oil—this will cause it to spread and enlarge the affected area. Redness or irritation may last 20 minutes to an hour.

- Never use oils undiluted on your skin. Always dilute with a carrier oil. If redness, burning, itching, or irritation occurs, stop using oil immediately. Be sure to wash hands after handling pure, undiluted essential oils.

- For sensitive skin or when using a new oil, perform a "Skin Patch Test." If irritation occurs, discontinue use of such oil or blend. See section, Skin Patch Test.

- If you are pregnant, lactating, suffer from epilepsy, have cancer, liver damage, or another medical condition, use essential oils under the care and supervision of a qualified Aromatherapist or medical practitioner.

- If taking prescription drugs, check for interaction between medicine and essential oils (if any) to avoid interference with certain prescription medications.

- To avoid contact sensitization (redness or irritation of skin due to repeated use of same individual oil) rotate and use different oils.

SKIN PATCH TEST

Certain essential oils can cause sensitization or an allergic reaction in some individuals. When using a new oil for the first time, you may want to perform a simple skin patch test on the inside of your arm or your chest. Place one drop of the essential oil into a carrier oil. Apply one drop on the skin and cover with a bandage. If skin becomes irritated and red, remove the bandage and immediately wash the area with soap and water. If after 12 hours no irritation has occurred, it is safe to use on the skin.

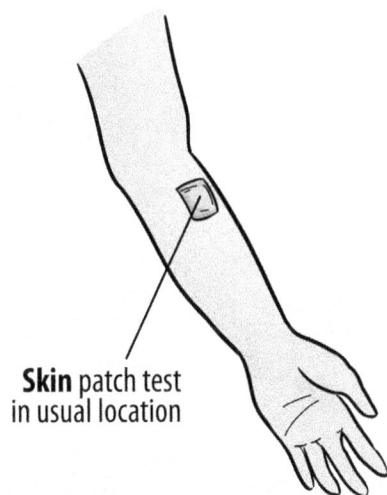

FIGURE. SKIN PATCH TEST

For someone who tends to be highly allergic, here is a simple test to determine if he or she is sensitive to a particular carrier oil and essential oil.

1. First, rub a drop of carrier oil onto the upper chest. In 12 hours, check for redness or other skin irritation.

2. If the skin remains clear, place 1 drop of selected essential oil in 15 drops of the same carrier oil, and again rub into the upper chest. If no skin reaction appears after 12 hours, it is safe to use the carriers and the essential oil.

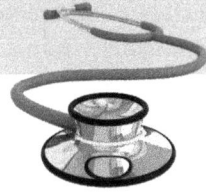

ESSENTIAL OILS
STORAGE

Because essential oils contain no fatty acids, they are not susceptible to rancidity like vegetable oils - but you will want to protect them from the degenerative effects of heat, light and air. Store them in tightly sealed, dark glass bottles away from any heat source. Properly stored oils can maintain their quality for years. (Citrus oils are less stable and should not be stored longer than six months after opening.)

ESSENTIAL OIL STORAGE TIPS:

- Keep oils tightly closed and out of reach of children.
- Always read and follow all labeled warnings and cautions.
- Do not purchase essential oils with rubber glass dropper tops. Essential oils are highly concentrated and will turn the rubber to a gum, thus ruining the oil.
- Make note of when the bottle of essential oil was opened and its shelf life.

- Many essential oils will remove furniture finish. Use care when handling open bottles.
- Keep essential oil vials and clear glass bottles in a box or another dark place for storing.

Be selective of where you purchase your essential oils. The quality of essential oil varies widely from company to company. Additionally, some companies may falsely claim their oils are undiluted and pure when they are not.

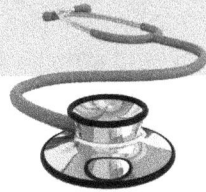

METHODS OF USE FOR
HIGH BLOOD PRESSURE

Various mechanisms can be used to deliver essential oils to target sites in the body. Common routes of administration include the skin and through inhalation. Essential oils may also be given orally and by rectal suppositories. Oral ingestion, however, is not recommended by many Aromatherapists since some essential oils available today can be harmful to the lining of the gut. For this reason, ingesting oils will not be addressed in this book due to the fact that some essential oils have also been known to cause liver and kidney damage when ingested. Regardless of which route of administration is used, the essential oils have to travel to the site of action with either the help of blood, nerves or oxygen (when inhalation route is used).

TOPICAL OR DERMAL

Through the skin, the essential oils get into the bloodstream where they travel to the target location. Massaging the skin can increase absorption of the oils. Some studies have suggested that areas of skin with a higher concentration of sweat glands and hair follicles have a higher rate of absorption including the soles of the feet, arms and armpits. Several research studies noted in this book advocate that soft-tissue massage does in fact reduce blood pressure.

GARGLE/MOUTHWASH

Add 3 drops of essential oil to 1 teaspoon of water to use as a mouthwash.

BATH

For a full bath, mix 8-10 drops of essential oil into two ounces of sea salts or a cup of milk then pour into a running bath. Agitate water in a figure eight motion to make sure the oil is mixed well, preventing irritation to mucous membranes.

Another method is to add essential oils after the bath has been drawn. Mix essential oils into a palm full of liquid soap, shampoo or a tablespoon of Jojoba oil and swish around to dissolve in the tub. Soak for 15-20 minutes.

SHOWER

While showering, add a drop or two of essential oil to a washcloth and rub on body.

MASSAGE

A variety of techniques used in massage therapy can incorporate the use of essential oils. Add 6-9 drops of essential oil to 1 Tablespoon of your favorite carrier oil to massage into body.

LOTIONS/CREAMS

Blending essential oils in an unscented, natural lotion/cream base allow you to benefit from the therapeutic qualities of the essential oil, giving you a non-oily way to apply essential oils. This is especially useful for someone with a skin condition that does not do well with oils. The dilution rate for using essential oils in a lotion base is no more than 2%. For adults, use 20 drops of essential oil to four ounces of lotion. For children and elderly, use 10 drops of essential oil to four ounces of lotion.

SPRAYS/SPRITZERS

Creating your own body sprays and facial mists is one of the easiest ways to use essential oils. For a facial mist, use 8-10 drops of essential oil in a four-ounce spray bottle filled with distilled water. For body sprays, add 20-30 drops of essential oil per four-ounce spray bottle filled with distilled water. For room sprays, use 40-60 drops of essential oil per four-ounce spray bottle with the remainder filled with distilled water.

BODY OILS

Mix 30 drops of essential oil per one ounce of cold-pressed carrier oil such as coconut oil. Choose an all-purpose oil that relieves stress and/or tension, headaches, and smells terrific.

INHALATION

Inhalation can be enhanced with the use of a nebulizer or a cool-mist diffuser in which essential oils are dispersed into the air. Other devices such as a light ring, vaporizer, or electric burner may be used instead, though heating oils may alter their molecular structure and can lose some of their effectiveness.

Inhalation is one of the easiest methods of use and is considered the most direct pathway for an aromatic blend or essence. When inhaled, fragrant vapors enter the lungs and are instantly released into the bloodstream for delivery to every cell in the body. Scientific research shows that essential oils can remain in a person's bloodstream for up to 4-6 hours, depending on the essential oil.

Essential oils that are properly diffused are known to kill bacteria and viruses, improve mental clarity, enhance or calm emotions, and increase feelings of well being. Over time, oils diffused can strengthen the immune system, reduce mold, and eliminate unpleasant odors. If a diffuser is not available, making a room spray, personal inhaler, or placing a few drops on a tissue to inhale will suffice. All are very effective ways to benefit from the healing properties of essential oils in the treatment of high blood pressure.

DIRECT INHALATION

Apply 2-3 drops of essential oils into your hand and rub palms together. Cup hands over the nose and mouth. Inhale vapors deeply several times.

HUMIDIFIER/VAPORIZER

For a humidifier or vaporizer, place 10 drops of essential oil undiluted into the unit.

LINENS/BLANKETS

Add your favorite essential oil to a spray bottle with water and spray to freshen bed sheets and blankets at bedtime and enhance deep sleep.

POTTERY/ELECTRIC BURNERS

A wide range of burners is available to use—some electric, some using tea light candles. Generally, tea light candles are not too hot for diffusing essential oils, but you may want to drop oils over glass stones or add water to the top part to help diffuse fragrance. Use caution around an open fire, as essential oils are flammable. Six drops of oil are recommended for everyday use; however, you may want to reduce the amount of oil used for rooms of the elderly or children.

NEBULIZER/DIFFUSER

Place 25 drops of essential oil undiluted inside the diffuser and use as needed. Limit diffusion of new oils to 10 minutes each day increasing the time until desired effects are reached. Adjust times for different-sized rooms and the strength of each fragrance. Unlike cheap fragrant oils purchased at department stores to mask odors, diffusing pure essential oils actually alters the structure of the molecules that create odors – rendering them harmless. Essential oils increase the available oxygen in the room and produce negative ions, which kill microbes.

QUICK REFERENCE BLENDING CHART

Here's a quick guide to use in determining how much essential oil to use for each application. For recipes and formulas, be sure to follow amounts listed in the directions. For children, elderly and pregnant women, please divide the essential oil amount in half for body applications.

Method	Carrier/Amount	Essential Oils Drops
Vaporizer	Full	5-10
Humidifier	Full	5-10
Steam Inhalation	Full Bowl	2-3
Diffuser/Nebulizer	-	10-25
Tea Lights/Burner	-	4-6
Room Spray	4 ounces	80-100
Body Lotion	4 ounces	25
Body Oil	4 ounces	50
Massage Oil	1 tablespoon	7-10
Shampoo	1 ounce	10
Conditioner	1 ounce	10
Chest Rub	1 ounce	15-25
Tissue	-	1-2
Mouthwash	1 teaspoon	2-3
Foot Bath/Spa	Small Tub	5
Bath	Full Tub	8-10
Shower	Washcloth	1-2

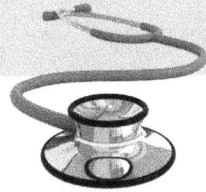

HOW TO USE ESSENTIAL OILS FOR TREATMENT OF HIGH BLOOD PRESSURE

There are several options available for controlling your blood pressure in both allopathic and alternative medicine. Many people today are able to regulate their blood pressure with the help of therapeutic quality essential oils along with a vigilance and commitment to a healthy diet and lifestyle.

In addition to the all the various methods of use listed in the previous chapter, two of the most effective methods for using essential oils for high blood pressure will be by inhalation and topically. Topically seems to be one of the most effective and favorite methods. For example, massage stimulates circulation of the blood while reducing muscular tension, aches, and pain. In addition, it significantly reduces stress and can offer comfort and peace of mind, allowing healing to take place. Inhalation of certain essential oils, on the other hand, helps to reduce stress as research has proven and is an effective ways to relax the body and calm the mind.

INHALATION

- Diffuse your choice of oils for ½ hour, three times a day. You may want to use one specific essential oil (with no carrier oil added) such as Jasmine, Neroli, or Lavender. Or, you may blend a combination of essential oils together.
- Place 2-3 drops of your chosen essential oil in your hand and rub your palms together. Cup hands over your nose and inhale deeply.
- Add 1-2 drops of essential oil to a tissue and carry with you to smell throughout the day or add several drops of pure essential oil to a pocket diffuser and use 2-3 times daily.

TOPICALLY

- Place essential oil on heart points on left arm, wrists, feet, and over heart.
- Rub 1-2 drops of essential oil on the temples and back of neck several times daily.
- Rub essential oil or essential oil blend on the bottom of feet each evening before bed.
- Massage an essential oil blend (with a carrier oil) for several minutes over the heart and carotid arteries along the neck. Be sure to monitor your blood pressure to see if it drops after massaging oils in. Reapply as desired.

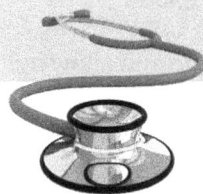

ESSENTIAL OIL
RECIPES FOR
HIGH BLOOD
PRESSURE

The following recipes are easy to make and simple to use. Keep in mind, though, because the root cause of high blood pressure is unknown, results may vary from person to person. You will want to experiment and try different essential oils to see which blend is right for you, as there is not one protocol that addresses every situation. You may choose to use one blend in the morning, and another at night. That's fine. Just remember to apply topical blends at least three times a day. The key points for application include the wrists, the feet, over the heart, on the carotidal arteries, and along the back of the neck.

The use of certain essential oils such as Lavender, Sweet Marjoram, and Ylang Ylang for helping to reduce high blood pressure can be very effective in relieving the stress and tension that may have attributed to the elevation of blood pressure. Other essential oils such as Roman Chamomile, Bergamot, Neroli, and Frankincense also help to bring harmony and create a more balanced terrain as a complementary treatment of high blood pressure. Feel free to experiment with different combinations of these oils and methods to find which one works best for you. Each oil contains unique and therapeutic qualities that can be beneficial for anyone suffering from hypertension. Simply inhale or massage one of these blends in and allow the healing properties to soothe and revitalize your soul.

SMART TIP: Some people add a drop or two of Lemon essential oil to their drinking water to help regulate their blood pressure.

BRIGHT AND EARLY TOPICAL BLEND

What You Will Need:

3 drops Lavender essential oil

2 drops Sweet Marjoram essential oil

1 drop Neroli essential oil

15ml Almond oil (or another carrier oil such as Apricot)

What to Do:

1. In a small glass bottle or container, add the essential oils.
2. Add the Almond carrier oil and shake to blend.
3. Gently rub several drops of the blend into the wrists, the feet, over the heart, along the carotidal arteries and along the back of the neck after showering in the morning.
4. Apply three times a day (if using this blend throughout the day).

TRANQUIL SLEEP TOPICAL BLEND

What You Will Need:

3 drops Bergamot essential oil

2 drops Frankincense essential oil

1 drop Ylang Ylang essential oil

15ml Apricot oil (or another carrier oil such as Almond)

What to Do:

1. In a small glass bottle or container, add the essential oils.
2. Add the Apricot carrier oil, replace cap and shake to blend.
3. Gently rub several drops of the blend into the wrists, the feet, over the heart, along the carotidal arteries and along the back of the neck after bathing in the evening before bed.
4. Apply three times a day (if using this blend throughout the day).

EVENING STEAM INHALATION BLEND

What You Will Need:

3 drops Bergamot essential oil

2 drops Lavender essential oil

1 drop Ylang Ylang essential oil

What to Do:

1. In a small bowl add steaming hot water.
2. Place 2-3 drops of essential oil blend into the water and stir to mix.
3. Place a towel over your head and inhale for three to five minutes.

HEART PLUS ROLL-ON BLEND

What You Will Need:

10 drops Ylang Ylang essential oil

10 drops Cypress essential oil

10 drops Marjoram essential oil

10 drops Lemon essential oil

10 ml Fractionated Coconut oil (or another carrier oil)

What to Do:

1. In a 10ml glass roll-on bottle, add the essential oils.
2. Fill the remaining space with the fractionated coconut oil. Shake to blend.
3. To use, roll the oil blend on the wrists, on the bottoms of the feet, along the neck and over the chest, two to three times a day.

BP ROLL-ON BLEND

What You Will Need:

10 drops Ylang Ylang essential oil

5 drops Cypress essential oil

5 drops Sweet Marjoram essential oil

5 drops Frankincense essential oil

10 ml Fractionated Coconut oil (or another carrier oil)

What to Do:
1.   In a 10ml glass roll-on bottle, add the essential oils.
2.   Fill the remaining space with the fractionated coconut oil. Shake to blend.
3.   To use, roll the oil blend on the wrists, on the bottoms of the feet, along the neck and over the chest, two to three times a day.

HEART BLEND

What You Will Need:

2 drops Sweet Marjoram essential oil

2 drops Helichrysum essential oil

2 drops Frankincense essential oil

10 drops Favorite carrier oil

What To Do:
1.   In a small bottle or container, add all essential oils.
2.   Fill the remaining space in the bottle with your favorite carrier oil. Shake to blend.
3.   Apply several drops to the bottoms of the feet and massage in. Rub several drops into the wrists, along the breastbone, along the carotidal arteries, and along the back of the neck.

HEART ESSENTIAL BLEND

What You Will Need:

3 drops Lemon essential oil

2 drops Ylang Ylang essential oil

1 drop Frankincense essential oil

10 drops Favorite carrier oil

What To Do:
1. In the palm of your hand, mix essential oils and carrier oil with your finger.
2. Rub blend into the chest and along the arms. Breathe in deeply.

ANGINA RELIEF BLEND

What You Will Need:
3 drops Lavender essential oil
3 drops Sweet Marjoram essential oil
3 drops Ylang Ylang essential oil
10 drops Favorite carrier oil

What To Do:
1. In the palm of your hand, mix essential oils and carrier oil with your finger.
2. Rub blend on the soles of your feet and along the carotidal arteries.

CALMING BLEND

This meditative blend soothes the mind and quiets the soul.

What You Will Need:
2 drops Lavender essential oil
2 drops Geranium essential oil
1 drop Sandalwood essential oil
½ cup Bath Salts (optional)

What To Do:
1. In a small bottle or container add essential oils. Stir to blend.
2. Add several drops of this blend to a running bath and swish to mix thoroughly in water. Or, mix with bath salts first and then add to a hot bath.
3. Relax and inhale the aromas, allowing the oils to penetrate the whole body.

ESSENTIAL FIVE BLEND

This blend offers a powerful punch to the cardiovascular system and boosts circulation.

What You Will Need:
6 drops Ylang Ylang essential oil
6 drops Helichrysum essential oil
4 drops Frankincense essential oil
4 drops Sweet Marjoram essential oil
4 drops Cassia essential oil
25 drops Coconut oil (or choose your favorite carrier oil from the directory)

What To Do:
1. In a small bottle or container, add all essential oils.
2. Fill the remaining space in the bottle with Coconut oil or another carrier oil. Shake to blend.
3. Apply several drops to the bottoms of the feet and massage in. Rub several drops into the wrists, along the breastbone, along the carotidal arteries, and along the back of the neck.
4. This blend may be added to bath salts and used in a bath, too.

LOVE MY HEART MASSAGE BLEND

Your heart is hard at work every second of every day for you. Take time to reciprocate your appreciation by offering support and nourishment with a massage using this blend.

What You Will Need:
4 drops Lavender essential oil
4 drops Ylang Ylang essential oil
1 drop Melissa essential oil
1 drop Neroli essential oil
1 ounce Favorite carrier oil

What To Do:
1. In a bottle or small container, add essential oils.
2. Fill the remaining space with carrier oil. Replace cap and shake to blend.

3. Massage into body or have a massage therapist apply the blend for you.
4. Use daily or as needed.

HEARTWARMING BATH BLEND

Part of your healing process requires slowing down and taking time for yourself. Slink down into a warm, relaxing bath and allow your body to absorb these essences of life.

What You Will Need:
3 drops Ylang Ylang essential oil
2 drops Clary Sage essential oil
1 drop Marjoram essential oil
½ cup Bath Salts (optional)

What To Do:
1. Stir essential oils into a running bath, or add to bath salts first.
2. Soak in the bath for 15-20 minutes. Repeat daily or as needed.

BP DIFFUSER BLEND

Make this essential oil blend ahead of time and have ready to use when life gets hectic. Add several drops to a cool-mist diffuser and run for 10-15 minutes twice daily.

What You Will Need:
15 drops Clary Sage essential oil
10 drops Lavender essential oil
6 drops Ylang Ylang essential oil
4 drops Sweet Marjoram essential oil
Airtight container

What To Do:
1. In a glass bottle, add all of the essential oils. Shake to blend.
2. Add several drops of the essential oil blend into a diffuser at work or in your home and run for 15 minutes in the morning and evening before bedtime. You can also inhale from the bottle to help induce calm.

EASY DOES IT BLEND

Use this blend to stop heart racing, smooth out muscle tissue, ease spasms and improve circulation.

What You Will Need:

2 drops Lavender essential oil

2 drops Marjoram essential oil

2 drops Cypress essential oil

2 drops Helichrysum essential oil

What To Do:

1. In a glass bottle, add all of the essential oils. Shake to blend.
2. Apply to the chest area around the heart and to the bottoms of the feet in the morning and in the evening.

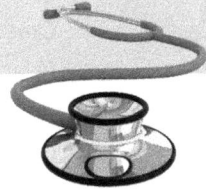

CREATING YOUR OWN BLENDS FOR
HIGH BLOOD PRESSURE

Creating your own essential oil blend for high blood pressure is easy to do when you follow the blend by note technique. Your essential oil blend will contain one or more oils from each of the following categories: Base note, Middle note and Top note (see chart below). Some apothecaries recommend using a fourth note, a fixative or bridge note such as Lavender, Chamomile, Marjoram or Vanilla. The bridge is what will help the other three oils blend together. Oftentimes Vitamin E oil is used.

The following chart contains essential oils that are known to be beneficial for high blood pressure. Each essential oil is listed by its common name and note classification: Top, Middle, and Base.

HYPERTENSION/HIGH BLOOD PRESSURE OILS

Top	Middle	Base
Bay Laurel	Blue Tansy	Cistus Labdanum
Bergamot	Cassia	Cypress
Clary Sage	Clove Bud	Frankincense
Garlic	Geranium	Ginger
Lemon	Ho Wood	Helichrysum
Oregano	Lavender	Jasmine
Neroli	Lavandin	Rose
Petitgrain	Marjoram	Spikenard
	Melissa	Turmeric
	Roman Chamomile	Valerian
	Yarrow	Ylang Ylang

Some oils made fall into more than one category. This is possible because of the many components essential oils possess and the synergy effect a blend might draw out of that oil. For this reason, you may find aromatherapists disagree to which group they fall in. However, don't let this trouble you. Instead, let this work to your advantage when creating your therapeutic blends. For instance, there may come a time when you have several middle note essential oils on hand to choose from, but no top notes for your specific condition. In this case, you could use an essential oil that may be a top note and middle note as your top note, and choose a different oil as your middle note.

Follow this simply as a guide when orchestrating your blends and let your nose have the final say.

TOP NOTES are oils that have a light, fresh aroma. It is the first scent you smell after applying a blend to the skin. Although they quickly evaporate, the top note is what gives us our first impression of a blend. Common top notes include Lemon, Bergamot, Orange, Lime and other citrus oils. In fact, Bergamot oil is one of the most widely essential oils used in the perfumery and toiletry industry, together with Neroli and Lavender, as the main ingredients for the classical Eau-de-cologne fragrance.

Most top notes are made up chemically of aldehydes and esters, which are generally found in oils from fruits, flowers and leaves.

For Blood Pressure Blends: Use 3 to 15 drops of a top note per 30 ml (or one ounce) carrier.

MIDDLE NOTES, also referred to as heart notes, are usually the inspiration for an aromatic blend or perfume and includes floral scents such as Roman Chamomile, Lavender, or Neroli. It is generally considered the heart of the blend as it often serves to cover up any unpleasant scents that may come from the base notes. Essential oils classified as middle notes are sometimes referred to as enhancers, equalizers, or balancers. Chemically, these are monoterpene alcohols found mostly in herbs and leaves. Examples of essential oil middle notes include Lavender, Roman Chamomile, Cypress, Geranium, Juniper Berry, Rosemary and Peppermint. Middle notes are what we smell when the scent from the top notes fades. This scent often evaporates after 15 seconds. The middle note can last 2-4 hours in the body and as the "heart" of the blend can play on the emotions. Middle notes are often found in flowers, leaves, and needles. They also act to bring together the top and base note as a "synergy" in a blend.

For Blood Pressure Blends: Use 2 to 10 drops of a middle note per 30 ml (or one ounce) carrier.

BASE NOTES, usually the backbone and foundation of the blend, is what the users will remember most about a particular fragrance. The scent of base notes will last the longest in the air and are what you smell after about 30 seconds of applying it to your skin. The base note is added to the mixture first. Examples of essential oil base notes include Vanilla, Sandalwood, Patchouli, Frankincense, Cinnamon, or other earthy and woodsy scents. Typically, a therapeutic blend has only one base note oil in it as it will stay the longest on the skin and can last up to 72 hours in the body. Aromatic blends can have one or more base oils to add character.

Chemically speaking, base notes are made up of sesquiterpenes or diterpenes and are mainly found in roots, gums and resins. Though therapeutic blends will typically contain one base note while aromatic blends may contain more than one, for any blend to be successful they must have a combination of all three notes.

For Blood Pressure Blends: Use 1 to 5 drops of a base note per 30 ml (or one ounce) carrier.

It is very important when making an essential oil blend for your high blood pressure to mix the extracts in order starting with the base note, followed by the middle note and finally the top note. This ensures your blend will create an aroma known as a "bouquet" by staying in tune with odor intensity as well as finding notes that strike a chord and harmonize well together in therapeutic properties.

It really is as easy as 1-2-3! Just remember, for every drop of base note, you add 2 drops of middle note and 3 drops of top note. This will ensure that your blood pressure blend is well-rounded having all three notes, and is chemically balanced between monoterpenes, sesquiterpenes and phenols.

MAKING YOUR FIRST BLOOD PRESSURE BLEND

Now that you have learned about how many drops of each note to use in your essential oil blend and have checked the precautions, it's time to start blending.

1. Before you begin, gather all of the necessary equipment: bottles, pipettes, essential oils, paper towels, labels, vials, and/or containers.

2. Make sure the counter space is clean and the area you are working in is well ventilated. You may want to put down wax paper (or a paper towel) to prevent any damage to the countertop from accidental spills. This will also make clean up much easier.

3. If you are using essential oils that are new to you, place one drop of the oil on a test strip (or small piece of paper) and wave it under your nose. Inhale the fragrance. If this fragrance is not what you had in mind for your blend, choose another oil and test again. You will want to do this with each oil until you have settled on the ones you want to use for your blend. It is a good idea to have a can of coffee grounds to smell after each fragrance to clear your palette.

4. Once, you have chosen the three oils for your blend, wave all three test strips fanned out beneath your nose and see if you like it. You may not care too much, as long as it helps lower your blood pressure, but keep in mind, if you despise the scent, you may be hesitant about using it regularly.

5. Check the safety precautions for the essential oils you have chosen to make sure there aren't any contradictions. Always take into consideration any other health conditions such as epilepsy, or any medications that may cause an adverse effect. The safety precautions must always be taken into consideration for the method you choose in their usage and for the person you are formulating the blend for.

6. Choose a new, clean bottle to use. Using a pipette, extract each essential oil into the bulb to place in your bottle. You may need to squeeze more than once

to get the amount you want. Remember to use a separate pipette or glass eye dropper for each of the oils used.

Add your base note essential oil first, one drop at a time. This is typically the most viscous or thickest oil. Next, add the middle note essential oil, followed by the top note essential oil. Be careful to use only the exact number of drops your recipe calls for. One drop too many can alter the results. Replace the cap on the bottle and shake to mix oils together.

7. Add your essential oil blend to a carrier oil (or lotion, gel, sea salts, etc.) and blend well to distribute the oils. What you use as your carrier and how much to add will depend on which method of application (Massage Blend, Bath Blend, Room Spray, etc.) you choose.

TIP: Always leave ½ inch of head space at the top of your bottle allowing your pure essential oil blend to breathe and expand.

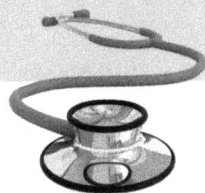

BASIC RECIPES FOR YOUR BLOOD PRESSURE BLENDS

Now that you have a basic understanding of how to blend essential oils together for high blood pressure, follow these simple recipes as a guideline for preparing your own products. You can formulate your own blend that will deliver the healing benefits you are seeking using three of the essential oils on the recommended list.

The recipes below are based on blending by notes. Of course, there is plenty of room for creativity as there are no hard and fast rules when it comes to creating your individual blend. You can add more or less. Feel free to change these to suit your own personal taste!

BASIC MASSAGE OIL BLEND RECIPE

Here is an easy-to-follow basic recipe for making a massage blend! You get to decide which essential oils to use depending on the type of massage and affect you looking to achieve.

What You Will Need:
1 ounce (30 ml) Carrier Oil, Lotion, or Gel
9-15 drops Top Note Essential Oil
6-10 drops Middle Note Essential Oil
3-5 drops Base Note Essential Oil
Plastic Bottle

What To Do:
1. Pour your carrier oil, lotion or gel into a clean bottle.
2. Add your essential oils one drop at a time, starting with your base note, followed by the middle note, and then the top note.
3. Shake well to mix oils and carrier together.
4. Add a label with name, ingredients and date created.
5. Use as normal.

BASIC BATH GEL BLEND RECIPE

Bath blends are easy to create using this basic recipe with a few essential oils!

What You Will Need:
1 teaspoon Glycerin, Gel, or Aloe Vera
3-12 drops Top Note Essential Oil
2-8 drops Middle Note Essential Oil
1-4 drops Base Note Essential Oil
Small Dish or Bowl

What To Do:
1. In a small dish or bowl, add the glycerin or gel as your fixative.
2. Add your essential oils one drop at a time to the fixative and stir well.
3. Pour your bath blend into a stream of warm running bath water. Enjoy!

BASIC BODY LOTION BLEND RECIPE

Do you want to try a good body lotion recipe? Why not make your own by following these simple instructions?

What You Will Need:
4 ounces Unscented Lotion, Hydrosol and/or carrier oil
18 drops Top Note Essential Oil
12 drops Middle Note Essential Oil
6 drops Base Note Essential Oil
Plastic Bottle or container

What To Do:
1. Place your carrier oil and/or lotion in your bottle.
2. Add essential oils starting with your base note essential oil first, followed by the middle note, and then the top note essential oil.
3. Recap and shake well to mix.
4. Use as normal.

BASIC LINEN SPRAY BLEND RECIPE

Use this special blend to ease insomnia and ensure better sleep at night. Don't forget when using essential oils for your spray to make sure the ones you choose are relaxing!

What You Will Need:
8 ounces Hydrosol, Floral Water, or Distilled Water
1 Tablespoon Glycerin
60 drops Top Note Essential Oil
40 drops Middle Note Essential Oil

20 drops Base Note Essential Oil

Glass or Plastic Spray Bottle

What To Do:

1. In a clean spray bottle, add the fixative (Glycerin).

2. Add your essential oil to the fixative, starting with the base note, followed by the middle note, and then the top note. Shake well.

3. Pour the Hydrosol or floral water into the bottle and shake to mix contents well.

4. Spray on bedspread and linens before making bed.

BASIC BATH SALTS BLEND RECIPE

For this basic bath salts recipe, you can use Dead Sea, Himalayan, or Epsom salts. Soak in a bath with this great blend to soothe away the stress of the day. Your bath salts can be made in advance and stored in a pretty container for convenience.

What You Will Need:

2 cups Epsom Salts

1 cup Sea Salts

1 cup Baking Soda

30 drops Top Note Essential Oil

20 drops Middle Note Essential Oil

10 drops Base Note Essential Oil

Wide Mouth Jar or container

What To Do:

1. In a container, add your essential oils starting with the base note, followed by the middle note, and then the top note. Stir to mix well.

2. Add sea salts and mix well to thoroughly saturate the salts with the oils.

3. In a running bath, add bath salts and swish around in the tub to mix thoroughly.

> **TIP:** Be sure to check precautions for oils that may cause sensitivity to skin. Not recommended for children.

BASIC SALT SCRUB BLEND RECIPE

Salt scrubs are great for increasing circulation. For this basic salt scrub recipe, you can choose which salt you prefer such as Dead Sea, Himalayan, or Epsom salts. Try it for painful joints and achy muscles, too. Your salt scrub can be made fresh each time, or you may want to make some up and store in a pretty container for when the time is right.

What You Will Need:
½ cup Sea Salts
2-4 ounces Carrier Oil (your choice)
9-12 drops Top Note Essential Oil
6-8 drops Middle Note Essential Oil
3-4 drops Base Note Essential Oil
Wide Mouth Jar or container

What To Do:
1. In a container, add your carrier oil, such as Almond or Coconut oil. Add your essential oils starting with the base note, followed by the middle note, and then the top note. Stir to mix well.
2. Add sea salts and mix well to thoroughly saturate the salts with the oils.
3. In the shower or bath, scrub the salt solution into the skin in upward motions toward the heart and in the direction of the lymph flow.

TIP: Be sure to check precautions for oils that may cause sensitivity to skin. Not recommended for children.

BASIC SALVE BLEND RECIPE

Carrying a small tin in your pocket is not only convenient but is easy to use.

What You Will Need:
½ - 1 cup Olive Oil or another Carrier Oil
2 teaspoons Beeswax
9 drops Top Note Essential Oil
6 drops Middle Note Essential Oil

3 drops Base Note Essential Oil

Small Jar or Tin

What To Do:

1. Using a glass double boiler, heat the oil over hot water. If you prefer, you can heat oil in a pan directly over the burner on low heat or in a microwave until warm.

2. Add the beeswax and stir until melted.

3. Let oil cool slightly (not too long or it will set up).

4. Add the essential oils, starting with the base note, followed by the middle note, then the top note. Stir to blend.

5. Pour mixture into jars or tins immediately. If mixture begins to set, just reheat slightly.

TIP: For variation, you can use solid Coconut oil and omit the beeswax. You may also want to add 6-8 Vitamin E oil capsules as a preservative.

BASIC BATH TEA BLEND RECIPE

For an extraordinary bathing experience, try adding dried herbs and flower petals to your running bath for a relaxing time!

What You Will Need:

2 cups Herbs (Lavender flowers, Mint leaves, etc.)

1 cup Sea Salts (your choice)

6 drops Top Note Essential Oil

4 drops Middle Note Essential Oil

2 drops Base Note Essential Oil

What To Do:

1. In a mixing bowl, add dried herbs and flower petals to sea salts and stir to blend.

2. Add essential oils starting with the base oil, followed by the middle note, then finally the top note. Stir to mix well.

3. Store in an airtight container or jar. Add a scoopful of mixture into a cotton or linen bag and hang under running bath water. If you do not have a bag, add mixture directly into bath. Enjoy!

BASIC BODY DETOX WRAP BLEND RECIPE

Body wraps are a popular way to lose weight and fight cellulite, which in turn helps lower blood pressure. In addition, you can kickstart your body's immune system by ridding yourself of accumulated chemicals and toxins stored in the body's lymphatic system.

What You Will Need:
3 ounces Distilled Water
12 drops Top Note Essential Oil
6 drops Middle Note Essential Oil
3 drops Base Note Essential Oil
Small glass Spray Bottle
Plastic Wrap

What To Do:
1. In a small spray bottle, add your essential oils starting with the base note, followed by the middle note, then the top note oil. Add the distilled water to the bottle, close and shake to blend.
2. Spray a bath towel thoroughly with the detox blend. Wrap the towel around your body, followed by tightly wrapping plastic wrap around yourself. Relax for 20 minutes before removing plastic wrap and towel.

BASIC ROLL-ON OIL BLEND RECIPE

This basic recipe can be used to create a roll-on bottle applicator for your essential oil blend, depending on the oils you have on hand. Keep track of what you add or change, so you'll know how to make your favorite blends at a later time.

What You Will Need:
½ Ounce Jojoba Oil
9 drops Top Note Essential Oil
6 drops Middle Note Essential Oil

3 drops Base Note Essential Oil
Dark Bottle

What To Do:
1. Add your carrier oil such as Jojoba to a clean, dark glass bottle.
2. When adding essential oils, start with the base note and then add the middle note, followed by the top note. As you add each one, check the scent to make sure it is what you are looking for.
3. Insert the ball insert and apply 2-3 times a day.

BASIC BATH OIL BLEND RECIPE

After a long day, soaking in a warm bath with a relaxing essential oil blend can be a sensual treat. Not only does it help take the edge off tense muscles, it ensures a better night's sleep. For early risers, starting your day with an invigorating essential oil blend at bath time may be more your speed, kickstarting your morning! Of course, a bath essential oil blend for achy joints can be helpful any time of day!

What You Will Need:
1 cup Almond Oil or Coconut Oil
30 drops Top Note Essential Oil
20 drops Middle Note Essential Oil
10 drops Base Note Essential Oil
Corked container
Crystal beads, dried flowers, small seashells, etc. (Optional)

What To Do:
1. Pour the carrier oil through a funnel into the corked container, leaving about an inch at the top.
2. When adding essential oils, start with the base note and then add the middle note, followed by the top note. As you add each one, check the scent to make sure it is what you are looking for.
3. Cork the container and agitate the bottle gently.
4. Let it sit for 2-3 days before using. Add decor to your bottle.
5. For use, pour ½ - 1 teaspoon into the palm of your hand and gently massage into the body after a bath.

BASIC NASAL INHALER BLEND RECIPE

Filling a blank nasal inhaler with your personal essential oil blend is an effective way to experience the therapeutic power of essential oils when suffering from high blood pressure or emotional issues. Inhalers are also great to use for colds, flu, headaches, allergies, lung and chest congestion. They are small enough to carry in a pocket or purse and have on hand for immediate relief. Add 15-18 drops of your essential oil blend to your inhaler.

What You Will Need:
9 drops Top Note Essential Oil
6 drops Middle Note Essential Oil
3 drops Base Note Essential Oil
Glass or Plastic Disposable Dropper
Small Plastic Inhaler

What To Do:
1. In a small bottle, add essential oils starting with the base oil, followed by the middle note, then finally the top note. Stir to mix well.
2. Use a glass or disposal dropper to fill nasal inhaler.
3. Carry and take a whiff as needed.

BASIC FOOT OIL BLEND RECIPE

A luxurious foot treatment with essential oils can readily deliver healing throughout the body. The sensitive skin and tissues of the feet take a lot of abuse and deserve a special blend that can easily be massaged in.

What You Will Need:
1 ounce (30ml) Almond Oil
3 drops Top Note Essential Oil
2 drops Middle Note Essential Oil
1 drop Base Note Essential Oil
Plastic or Glass Bottle

What To Do:

1.   In a glass or plastic bottle, add your essential oils starting with the base note, followed by the middle note and then the top note. Mix well.

2.   Add the Almond oil or another carrier oil to the bottle, replace lid and shake to blend.

3.   To use, massage oil blend into feet after a bath or shower, or before bed. Wear soft, cotton socks to bed.

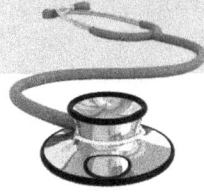

WHICH CARRIER OILS TO USE WHEN CREATING TOPICAL BLENDS

When you use essential oils on the skin, in most cases you will want to dilute with a carrier or vegetable oil. Carrier oils come from nuts, seeds or kernels that contain essential fatty acids, fat-soluble vitamins, minerals and other crucial nutrients. You will find a variety of carrier oils to choose from, each possessing different therapeutic properties.

The two main methods of producing carrier oil are cold-pressed and maceration. These processes ensure they have not been modified by heat, which would destroy the vital nutrients contained in the oil, and are as natural and unadulterated as possible.

Macerated oils, such as calendula and carrot oils, are made from a combination of base oil such as sunflower and plant material that has been left in an airtight container over a period of time in order to infuse the liquid with the plant's constituents.

Carrier oils and infused oils are used to dilute essential oils and absolutes by offering the necessary lubrication and moisture to the skin for aromatherapy. Distinct from essential oils, carrier oils do not contain aromatic scents (or only a very faint scent) and evaporate due to their large molecular structure. For this reason, most consider carrier oils just a vehicle for applying essential oils to the skin in massage. However, they do offer their own healing properties in which essential oils do not possess. Your aromatherapy experience can be significantly enhanced by choosing the best combination of carrier and essential oils.

Consultant Nancy Jackson of Ananda Aromatherapy, an online source for therapeutic aromatherapy techniques and supplies, writes, "Many carrier oils can be used in multiple applications, and consumers often choose oils based on the thickness or scent they prefer. Individual carrier oils do have some specific qualities, though, that can be used to your benefit.

"The main carrier oils used today are determined by their common aromatherapy application. Sweet Almond, Sunflower, Hempseed, and Fractionated Coconut are excellent choices for massage and reflexology. A mixture of 10-15% essential oil and 85-90% carrier oil will ensure a powerful massage oil that is smooth and great-smelling.

"When choosing your own carriers, experiment with a few and see how your skin responds. Once you find one you love (and there's definitely a carrier oil for everyone) you can begin mixing the carrier with your favorite essential oils."

SHELF LIFE OF CARRIER OILS

A carrier oil's shelf life, which is the length of time before a particular oil begins to turn rancid, can be greatly influenced by heat and light. You will want to store your oils in a cool, dark place to preserve their freshness, and in some cases refrigerate (e.g. Not Avocado), as heat and sunlight can shorten their shelf life. When refrigerating, oils may appear cloudy but will regain their clear state upon returning to room temperature. If you have a large amount of carrier oil on hand, you can freeze the unused portion until ready for use.

TIP: Try not to mix too much of your favorite massage blend in advance if you don't plan on using it right away.

Carrier Oil	Shelf Life
Fractionated Coconut	Indefinite
Flaxseed	3–6 months
Grapeseed	3–6 months (up to 9 months, if refrigerated)
Olive	12–18 months
Sweet Almond	12 months
Jojoba	Indefinite
Apricot Kernel	6–12 months
Argan	24 months
Avocado	12 months
Borage	6 months
Carrot Seed	12 months
Cocoa Butter	3–5 years
Coconut (virgin)	2–4 years
Cranberry Seed	2 years
Evening Primrose	6–12 months
Hemp Seed	12 months
Macadamia	12 months
Palm	24 months
Pomegranate Seed	12 months
Rosehip Seed	6 months
Safflower	12 months
Walnut	12 months
Pumpkin Seed	6–12 months
Meadowfoam Seed	Indefinite
Wheat Germ	1 year

Joline Alta, Co-founder of http://AnandaApothecary.com, writes, "Carrier oils do follow on the coattails of the exotic repertoire of essential oils. This category includes any plant-derived oil that primarily functions as a base oil for containing, delivering and enhancing an essential oil. While essential oils are short-chain molecules that quickly dissolve when exposed to air (thus the term 'volatile oils,' meaning quick to change), carrier oils are longer-chain molecules that do not break down as rapidly and hold their shape and qualities longer.

"Essential oils and carrier oils have a symbiotic relationship in aromatherapy. While carriers are often thought of in terms of their reflexology and massage uses, these oils actually possess their own virtues. Instead of thinking of them as merely the method of applying essential oils, we can explore the unique qualities of carrier oils separately with impressive results. Most likely, your aromatherapy techniques will be enhanced by using your specific essential oils with carriers that actually increase their medicinal qualities.

"To begin with, it is important to remember that fats are essential for human life. Fats, called lipids, are critical for maintaining warmth, providing protection and ensuring healthy cellular function. Although the world of nutrition is engaged in discovering which fats are best for internal health, aromatherapy is concerned with how plant-derived oils deliver health from the outside in. Externally applied oils help the body maintain vital functions in unique ways through both chemical changes and mechanical assistance.

"Fat molecules are composed of hydrogen, oxygen and carbon atoms. It's easy to become immediately confused when chemistry comes into the mix, but because so many of these fat buzz words are found in natural health and nutrition, it's useful to understand where the aromatherapy carrier oils fall in the spectrum of lipids. A basic explanation of fat composition is that while all fats contain carbon atoms, some fats have carbon atoms that are double bonded to one another, meaning they share electrons. These fats are called unsaturated fats; they are liquid at room temperature and they are derived from vegetables.

"Most carrier oils are unsaturated fats. Saturated fats have carbon bonds that do not bind to other carbon atoms. These oils are solid at room temperature and include animal-derived fats and some plant-derived fats as well. Coconut oil is a saturated fat that is often used as a carrier oil. Fractionated coconut, another common carrier oil, occurs when a coconut molecule has been altered to keep it in a liquid, rather than solid, state. The healing qualities of the oil are not compromised and we can use the oil the same way we'd use a seed or nut oil.

"Many carrier oils have the essential fatty acids Omega-6 (linoleic acid) and Omega-3 (linolenic). Essential fatty acids must be acquired through outside sources, primarily through diet, and are critical to maintaining health. According to Aromatherapist Salvatore Battaglia, Omega-6, which is vital for skin, hair, liver function, joints, healing wounds and circulation, is especially powerful in Evening Primrose oil, a popular and versatile carrier oil. Omega-3 is also in many carrier oils. Taken internally, it helps with vision, muscles, and growth. It is found in fish and some vegetable oils, like linseed and canola. It is known to help circulation, assist in heart health, lower cholesterol and blood pressure, and prevent inflammation. The most important thing to remember about lipid structure in carrier oils is that choosing high-quality nutritious oils will significantly assist in its vital functions. Since the skin is the largest organ in the body and often needs assistance in maintaining its elasticity, vitality and moisture, carrier oils are truly the skin's best friend.

"Carrier oils are primarily derived from nuts and seeds. They are extracted via cold-pressed technology, meaning high heat is not used. Once oils reach temperatures exceeding 160 degrees Celsius, their structure is altered, making them trans-fats, a kind of mutated fat that the body cannot assimilate properly. Expeller-pressing is another common extraction method. By placing seeds or nuts in an expeller, the precious oil is pressed out and then bottled. Superior carrier oils are mechanically pressed oils and have not been subjected to chemical changes.

"There are many reasons for choosing one carrier oil over another, and most of the time this is based on personal preference regarding the viscosity of the oil and its natural scent. While this is a fine way to choose oils, if you want to include the specific healing benefits of carrier oils in your aromatherapy applications, it might be useful to look at how carrier oils are sometimes categorized.

"When carrier oils are used with essential oils, they provide a mechanism for the volatile oils to be transported more effectively. Most essential oils when applied externally move through the body system in an hour. A carrier oil, which is thicker than a volatile oil, "holds" the essential oil in place, delivering longer-lasting healing.

"Think of it this way: if you apply a drop of Lavender directly to your skin, within a relatively short period of time, the scent will dissipate. If you place the same amount of Lavender in a carrier oil and rub the carrier oil into the same spot, you will experience the scent longer.

"When we apply the same method for healing purposes, rather than simply attempting to make the scent last for aesthetic reasons, we can increase the healing power of an essential oil by ensuring it maintains contact with the body for a longer period of time.

"Since consistent application of essential oils over a period of time increases the healing potential of the oil, carrier oils help us keep the essential oil active once it touches the skin. Also, many essential oils are too harsh for direct contact with the skin, but once mixed with carriers, they cause no trouble whatsoever, and their healing potential is maximized.

"Carrier oils are certainly the least glamorous oils in the aromatherapy world, but with a little effort, these humble oils can bring a world of comfort from the outside in."

Essential oils in aromatherapy are highly concentrated and potent. Although there are only a few exceptions to using essential oils 'neat' or undiluted (such as Lavender and Chamomile), it is ideal to always use a carrier oil with your essential oils to avoid having an adverse effect or skin irritation.

Carrier oils provide the much-needed lubrication, allowing hands to move freely over the skin, helping with the absorption of essential oils into the body. Choose a carrier oil that is light, non-sticky and that can effectively penetrate the skin. Always check the label to make sure its 100% pure, unrefined and cold-pressed.

CARRIER OILS DIRECTORY

With the wide selection of carrier oils, each with various therapeutic benefits, choosing one will depend on the area it's being applied to, the treatment plan, and any skin sensitivities. When using an oil for massage, viscosity is an important consideration. Some carrier oils may work better than others in certain applications. For example, Grapeseed oil is generally very thin while Olive oil is much thicker, and others such as Sunflower and Sweet Almond have viscosities halfway between these extremes. You can easily blend carrier oils to combine their properties of viscosity, absorption rate, and benefits. Don't forget to take into consideration the color of your carrier oil when creating a special recipe where it may affect the outcome of the product; otherwise, for general blending purposes the color of your carrier oil won't matter.

TIP: When shopping for a good quality carrier oil, be sure it's cold-pressed so that all of its natural qualities have been retained.

ALMOND OIL is one of the most useful, practical and moderately priced carrier oils available. It is great for all skin types as it moisturizes and reconditions the skin with its satiny smooth texture. This pale yellow oil quickly absorbs into the skin, leaving your skin feeling soft and non-greasy. Sweet Almond provides relief from itching, soreness, dryness, inflammation, and is especially beneficial for eczema. As a lightly nutty refined oil rich in fatty acids, proteins and Vitamin D, it is everyone's favorite massage base oil for loosening stiff muscles and achy joints.

Dilution: Can be used at 100%.

APRICOT KERNEL OIL is pale yellow in color and has a light texture, is easily absorbed and moisturizes both the body and face well. Extracted from the kernel of apricot fruit, it contains Vitamin E, which is particularly good for mature skin. Vitamins A and B help in healing and rejuvenating skin cells. It is good for all skin types, especially for sensitive, inflamed and dry skin. Apricot seeds are well known for the presence of amygdalin, as well as Vitamin B-17 and laetrile, which is a compound considered to have the potential to kill cancer cells without causing any damage to surrounding healthy cells, and lower blood pressure. Studies reveal that the consumption of apricot seeds helped in the lowering of both systolic and diastolic blood pressure in people with high blood pressure.

Dilution: Can be used at 100% or as a blend with other carrier oils such as Sweet Almond oil for a massage at 10% dilution.

ARGAN OIL comes from Morocco with over 80% unsaturated fatty acids and essential fats. It contains high amounts of Vitamin E and is extremely resistant to oxidation. This cold-pressed oil is considered a treat for mature skin and valued for its nutritive, cosmetic and medicinal properties. Researchers have concluded daily consumption of Argan oil can help prevent various cancers, cardiovascular disease and obesity. According to the British Journal of Nutrition n (2004), 92, 921–929, "Argan (Argania spinosa) oil lowers blood pressure and improves endothelial dysfunction in spontaneously hypertensive rats." Its medicinal uses also include rheumatism and healing burns. Argan oil is sometimes mixed with Pomegranate Seed oil due to its anti-oxidizing properties.

Dilution: Can be used at 100% or diluted with other carrier oils such as Rosehip Seed, Coconut or Apricot Kernel as a blend.

AVOCADO OIL is rich in lecithin, Vitamins, A, B1, B2, D, and E. It also contains amino acids, sterols, pantothenic acid, and lecithin. It is known to delay aging as it is rich in essential fatty acids. Avocado easily penetrates the skin, acts as sunscreen and helps in cell regeneration. For skin that has been exposed to the sun, mix zinc oxide in half a bottle of Avocado oil and apply. Avocado is greatly praised for those who suffer with skin problems such as eczema, psoriasis, and other skin disorders. The antioxidants and beta-sitosterol found in avocados help to reduce the risk of heart disease and cancer, while maintaining eye health in aging adults. Avocados are also rich in monounsaturated fats, which help balance cholesterol levels. An essential nutrient for bone and cardiovascular health, the magnesium found in an avocado is also known to reduce migraines and prevent type II diabetes. The Omega-3 Fatty Acids in avocados may reduce inflammation, high cholesterol, high blood pressure, depression and arthritis.

Dilution: Can be used at 100%, although in most cases, it is best mixed with another carrier oil such as Sweet Almond or Grapeseed oil to make up 10-30% of the carrier blend.

BORAGE SEED OIL is naturally one of the greatest sources of GLA or gamma-linolenic acid. It improves the skin texture when used topically. Borage Seed is excellent for use with children with atopic dermatitis. During the Middle Ages, borage was a popular anti-inflammatory agent used to treat rheumatism and heart disease.

Dilution: Can be used at 100% as your carrier oil base, although it is recommended to use with other carrier oils up to 25% for therapeutic uses.

CARROT SEED OIL is rich in beta carotene and Vitamins A, B, C, D and E. This oil is known to heal dry, chapped skin, balance the moisture in skin and condition the hair, as well. It is suitable for all skin types, especially for dry, mature skin, and is effective for face and neck treatments in reducing wrinkles. Many users find it helpful for burns, wounds, cuts and scars. Carrot Seed oil contains up to 13 percent alpha-pinene and up to 18 percent carotol. Other contents include daucol, limonene, beta-bisabolene, eugenol, vanillin, various terpenoids, coumarin, and palmitic and butyric acids. The website Drugs.com credits Carrot Seed oil with smooth-muscle relaxant action, as well as the ability to protect the liver, dilate blood vessels and lower blood pressure in animal studies. Carrot Seed absorbs easily into the skin and is great for eczema, psoriasis, and itchy scalp.

Dilution: Can be used at 100% or blended with another carrier oil at 10-25%.

COCOA BUTTER is a rich and creamy butter (not a carrier oil) that must be warmed to make it liquid. It is a wonderful addition to skin care products due to its high level of polyphenols, vitamins and nutrients. It smoothes, hydrates, and balances skin while providing collagen to support mature skin. Its warm aroma of cocoa is a delightful addition in lotions and creams. Cocoa butter is widely used as a treatment for pregnancy stretch marks. With its A, B1, B2, B3, C, and E vitamins, it is an excellent moisturizer for skin health. Scientists have linked the cocoa (in dark chocolate and cocoa butter) to a reduction of blood pressure and heart disease. According to the American Heart Association, a 2006 study called "Circulation: Heart Failure" reported that middle-aged and elderly women who regularly ate a small amount of chocolate had a 32 percent lower risk of heart failure. Although scientists are not sure why, it may be due to its oleic acid or its cocoa mass polyphenol (CMP), which may protect against heart disease.

Dilution: Its solid texture makes it difficult to work in and needs to be blended with other oils to be workable. Use at a 10% dilution.

COCONUT OIL (FRACTIONATED) seems to be quickly becoming the carrier oil of choice because of its vast use in alternative medicine and healing. While it is fractionated, no change has been made chemically. Rather, its molecular structure 'fraction' has been separated, allowing it to remain liquid at room temperature making it much more useful in aromatherapy. Coconut oil is perfect as a moisturizer for the body and conditions brittle, dry or dull hair. Because of its many health benefits, Coconut oil, when used properly, can prove beneficial in a regimen designed to lower blood pressure. Its light, easily absorbable texture gives skin a smooth satin effect with virtually no scent of its own and an indefinite shelf life. Coconut oil is 92% saturated fat and contains Omega-3 fatty acids, and is believed to be better for lowering blood pressure than other vegetable oils. Omega-3 fatty acids are known to widen your blood vessels and relieve inflammation of the arteries.

Dilution: Can be used at 100%.

COCONUT OIL (VIRGIN) has an unbelievable balance of natural saturated fatty acids with antibacterial and antiviral properties not found in other oils. Coconut oil is perfect as a skin conditioner for nearly all skin conditions and is believed to stimulate hair growth. It has a light, aromatic coconut scent that becomes solid at room temperature. For this reason, it is recommended to blend with other carrier oils in your body care products. It is fully digestible and is considered a healthy cooking oil. Several virgin coconut oils are high in antioxidants which are positively associated with reducing oxidative stress, and thus lowering blood pressure.

Dilution: Can be used alone directly but is recommended to use 10-25% dilution with other carrier oils.

CRANBERRY SEED OIL is rich in Vitamin E and A, Omega-3, 6, and 9 fatty acids not available in other carrier oils. This fruity medium texture oil can help reduce signs of aging and heal scars and skin conditions such as eczema and psoriasis. Cranberries are high in antioxidants that help fight free radicals. The oil from the cranberry seed contains high levels of polyunsaturated and monounsaturated fatty acids, phospholipids, phytosterols and large amounts of antioxidants that offer a variety of health benefits. Cranberries are a good source of phenolic phytochemicals, including phenolic acids. According to an article published in the November 2007 issue of Nutrition Reviews, "Polyphenols found in cranberries may reduce the risk of cardiovascular disease by impeding platelet aggregation, lowering blood pressure and promoting resistance of low-density lipoprotein, or LDL, against oxidation."

Dilution: Can be used at 100%.

EVENING PRIMROSE OIL makes a delightful addition to your carrier oil blends. It is the perfect, lightly refined oil that can be used to moisturize, soften and soothe away dry and irritated skin and help with premature aging. Evening primrose contains gamma-linolenic acid, Omega-3 essential fats as well as other fatty acids that help the body produce prostaglandin E1, which reduces inflammation and improves digestion. Because evening primrose oil contains Omega-6 essential fatty acids that are necessary for good health, it has been known to lower blood pressure. This oil can be taken internally. Please note this oil can go rancid quickly.

Dilution: Due to its cost, it is usually blended with other carrier oils at 10% dilution.

FLAXSEED OIL is an emollient, high in essential fatty acids, Vitamin E, B, and minerals. It contains the alpha-linoleic acids (ALAs), which may contribute to lowering blood pressure. Flaxseed is reputed as being an excellent treatment for eczema and psoriasis. It is also known for its anti-inflammatory properties and for preventing scarring and stretch marks. Flaxseed oil contains both Omega-3 and Omega-6 fatty acids, which are needed for health. Flaxseed oil contains the essential fatty acid alpha-linolenic acid (ALA), which the body converts into eicosapentaenoic acid (EPA) and docosahexaenoic acid (DHA), the Omega-3 fatty acids found in fish oil according to the University of Maryland Medical Center's website. ALA may reduce heart disease risks through a variety of ways, including making platelets less "sticky," reducing inflammation, promoting blood vessel health, and reducing risk of arrhythmia (irregular heart beat). Several human studies also suggest that diets rich in Omega-3 fatty acids (including ALA) may lower blood pressure. This golden oil will leave a greasy feeling to the skin, so it is recommended to add to other carrier oils for use in skincare products.

Dilution: Due to its heavy scent and texture, use at 10% dilution with another carrier oil or carrier oil blend.

GRAPESEED OIL is a pleasing, light green and odorless oil, good as a base oil for many creams, lotions and as a carrier oil. Grapeseed oil is pressed from the seeds of a grape and contains OPCs, flavonoids, vitamin E, resveratrol, and fatty acids. It is non-allergenic and has very high levels of linoleic acid, with traces of proanthrocyanidins, which are very potent antioxidants. It is reportedly helpful to reduce stretch marks. It is used as an alternative treatment for conditions such as diabetes, hemorrhoids, cancers, high cholesterol, edema, and high blood pressure. A study conducted at the University of California at Davis found that grape seed extract helped control blood pressure. It is especially beneficial for all skin types because of its natural non-allergenic properties. Grapeseed works well, especially when other oils do not absorb well, without leaving a greasy feeling after application. Slightly astringent, it tightens and tones the skin and alleviates acne. Grapeseed makes an ideal carrier oil for body massage bases. Saturation takes longer than some other carrier oils.

Dilution: Can be used at 100%.

HEMP SEED OIL is a hidden treasure of fatty acids, including ALA and GLA, that makes it possibly one of the most nourishing oils available. An analysis shows it contains linoleic acid, Alpha and gamma linolenic Acid (omega-6), palmitic acid, Stearic acid and oleic acid. These essential fatty acids help ward off various age-related diseases and osteoarthritis. Hemp oil has been scientifically proven to improve dermatitis symptoms, reduce blood clots and high blood pressure. Like Evening Primrose, it is supportive of reducing inflammation, which makes it useful for arthritis and autoimmune disorders. It also stimulates hair and nail growth and makes a superb skin moisturizer. Hemp oil contains many healing and regenerative properties and may be applied topically to restore vital organs, as well as skin conditions. Research shows it is beneficial in reducing blood clots and high blood pressure. This rich, slightly green, nutty flavored oil can be taken internally but should be refrigerated.

Dilution: Can be used at 100% or blended with other carrier oils at 20% dilution for massage purposes.

JOJOBA OIL is bright and golden in color and is known as one of the best oils (really a liquid wax) for hair and skin. It penetrates the skin quickly and is excellent for skin nourishment and for healing inflamed skin, psoriasis, eczema, or any sort of dermatitis. Jojoba controls acne and oily skin, and makes a terrific scalp cleanser as excess sebum dissolves in Jojoba. It is good for all skin types and promotes a healthy, glowing complexion by gently unclogging the pores and lifting embedded impurities. It makes a good base oil for treating rheumatism and arthritis because of its anti-inflammatory actions. Jojoba is suitable for all aromatherapy uses other than a full-body massage. And, because of the oil's antioxidants, it does not become rancid and can even prevent rancidity in other oils.

Dilution: Can be used at 100% but due its price, many use a 10% dilution with other carrier oils.

MACADAMIA OIL has a rich golden color with mild nutty undertones. It is made up of 80% mono-unsaturated fatty acids including oleic acid, Palmitoleic acid, linoleic acid and linolenic acid. This oil's fatty acid closely resembles human sebum and a recent study show that the present of palmitoleic acid plays an active role in the slowing down of lipid peroxidation, thus offering cell protection function. Macadamia provides the skin with a silky feel and is quickly absorbed leaving a smooth, non-greasy feeling. Studies by the Journal of Nutrition revealed that consumption of macadamia nuts lowers plasma total and LDL cholesterol levels in hypercholesterolemic men. It is sensitive to light and will go rancid as a result. Use this oil in small quantities as the scent may overpower the blend.

Dilution: Use at 10-25% dilution with another carrier oil or carrier oil blend.

MEADOWFOAM SEED OIL with its pale yellow color and medium viscosity makes a nice carrier for many aromatherapy applications. Its rejuvenating properties make it a popular choice for cosmetics and skin care products especially for its UV protection properties. It is a key ingredient in many different products such as suntan lotion, massage oils and lotions, hand/facial creams, hair and scalp products, cuticle repair cream, foundations, rouges, face powders, lipsticks, shampoos, and shaving creams. Its rich antioxidant content of Vitamin E, oleic acid (Omega-9 fatty acid), erucic acid, ecosenoic acid, linoenic acid (Omega-6 fatty acid), delta linolenic acid and alpha Omega-3 fatty acids makes it a highly stable oil with an indefinite shelf life. At closer examination, the seed contains useful components such as tocopherol, the primary component of Vitamin E that is known to keep the skin from aging, protects different organs of the body and slows down its degeneration. It also contains docosadienoic acid, which is a polyunsaturated fat known for the benefits that it gives to the heart. Specifically, it can lower cholesterol and triglycerides in the body as well as lower blood pressure.

Dilution: Can be used at 10% dilution with another carrier oil or carrier oil blend.

OLIVE OIL (Extra Virgin) is light to medium green in color, with a rather heavy texture. It is very soothing and carries disinfecting and healing properties. Olive oil is quite legendary since it has been used over the centuries for multiple purposes, but due to its overpowering scent this oil does not work well for massages. However, it is beneficial in some lotions for burns or scars. Olive is very beneficial for dry, damaged or split hair and is soothing for inflamed skin such as eczema. It has been proven to be very beneficial for rheumatic conditions and protects the body against harmful free-radical cell damage. Traditionally, olive oil has been used for stomach disorders, stimulates bile production, promotes pancreatic secretions and may even protect against stomach ulcers. The anti-hypertensive effects of olive oil are so powerful many users eliminated their need for blood pressure-lowering medications in just six months, according to a recent study. The "virgin" indicates it comes from the first pressing of the fruit. The "extra" means it comes from a single source. Extra virgin olive oil is particularly good for high blood pressure because it contains more vitamin E than virgin, pure or extra light varieties. Historically, olive oil has been the base for anointing oils. Olive oil is commonly used in body lotions, soaps and hair products.

Dilution: Can be used at 100% or 25-50% dilution with another carrier oil blend.

PALM OIL comes from the fruit of the palm tree that is rich in palmitic acid, Vitamin E, Vitamin K and magnesium. Palm oil contains saturated and unsaturated fats, vitamin E, and beta-carotene. It has antioxidant effects and is used by many to lower blood pressure. Red palm oil has recently been studied for its beneficial role in fighting heart disease and high cholesterol. Dr. Oz's website states, "...studies show that adding palm oil into the diet can remove plaque build-up in arteries and, therefore, reverse the process of plaque and prevent blockages. In fact, studies funded by the National Institutes of Health (NIH) have shown that a natural form of vitamin E called alpha tocotrienol, which is the form found in high amounts in red palm fruit oil, can help reduce the effects of stroke by 50% by protecting your brain's nerve cells." In addition, red palm oil can improve cholesterol values and helps to maintain proper blood pressure. It is semi-solid at room temperature and must be warmed to become liquid. It is a natural source of antioxidants and is great for soap making.

Dilution: Can be used at 100% or 10% dilution with another carrier oil or carrier oil blend.

POMEGRANATE SEED OIL is highly sought after for beauty and skin care products. Rich in phytosterols, it is considered a treasure trove of beneficial properties for the skin because of its antioxidants, punicic acids and egallic acids. Punicic acid is an oil known as "Super CLA" or linoleic acid that is found to support healthy fat metabolism and weight loss. The oil is an excellent base for all types of skin conditions, including eczema, sunburn, dry and cracked skin and mature skin. Pomegranate Seed oil also revives the skin's elastic nature. Research has shown the oil to actually stimulate keratinocyte production, strengthening the dermis. Punicalagin, a compound found only in pomegranates, is shown to benefit the heart and blood vessels and is the major component responsible for pomegranate's antioxidant and health benefits. It not only lowers cholesterol, but also lowers blood pressure and increases the speed at which heart blockages (atherosclerosis) melt away, according to research. In other studies, potent antioxidant compounds found in pomegranates have shown to reduce platelet aggregation and naturally lower blood pressure, preventing both heart attacks and strokes. The oil is rich in phytoestrogens as well, which helps women manage menopause symptoms. Pomegranate Seed oil can be used alone or combined with a lotion or base oil such as Jojoba, Almond or Olive and then applied to the skin.

Dilution: Can be used at 100% or blended with another carrier oil at 25-50% dilution.

PUMPKIN SEED OIL is a mildly rich yellow oil, containing protein, oleic acid, linoleic acid, palmitic acid, Stearic acid, Omega-3 and Omega-6 fatty acids, which are known to support brain function, and give you overall health and vitality. Pumpkin Seed oil also contains high levels of Vitamin E, as well as Vitamins A and C, Zinc, and other trace minerals and vitamins. This oil strengthens the lungs and mucous membranes, and can be used as an alternative to fish oils. It is useful as a diuretic for urinary complaints, as a demulcent and as an anthelmintic to expel intestinal worms. It is readily absorbed by the skin and can be used by all skin types. Pumpkin Seed oil is fabulous for combating fine lines and makes a great moisturizer for face creams, lotions, bath oils, massage oils and other skincare products.

Dilution: Use at a 10% dilution with another carrier oil or carrier oil blend.

ROSEHIP OIL is called the queen of carrier oils because of its luxurious treatment for wrinkles, scars and inflamed skin. It is a good oil for cosmetic uses as it helps with cell regeneration by preventing premature aging and smoothing lines. In addition, Rosehip is good for eczema, psoriasis, PMS, menopause and high blood pressure. According to a study conducted and published in the European Journal of Clinical Nutrition, supplements with Rosehip significantly reduced blood pressure and LDL cholesterol. Cold-pressed from the seeds of Rosehips, its pale yellow light texture makes it a wonderful carrier oil for skin care.

Dilution: Use sparingly alone, or use at 10% dilution when blended with other carrier oils.

SAFFLOWER OIL has a slight nutty aroma and is rich in Omega-6 group of essential fatty acids, oleic acid, palmitic acid, linoleic acid and linolenic acid as well as Vitamin E. It has the highest percentage of unsaturated fats of all vegetable oils. Because of its light texture, Safflower oil is suitable for body massage. It has diuretic properties and is helpful for painful inflamed joints, bruises and sprains. This oil is also great for skin allergies and is beneficial for people who suffer from arteriosclerosis and is a good choice for those who want to improve the health of their cardiovascular system. This oil oxidizes quickly. Safflower can be used in massage blends.

Dilution: Can be used at 100% or diluted with another carrier oil blend.

SESAME OIL has a rich golden color with a bold, nutty flavor. It is a warm oil that is used for conditions such as eczema, psoriasis and arthritis. Sesame oil is active with Vitamin A and E, minerals and lecithin. Research has shown Sesame oil enriches the blood, stimulates the blood platelet count, and is effective against spleen disorders. One website reported, "It is almost as effective as a drug for bringing down high blood pressure, and the oils also improve cholesterol levels." It is high in calcium and makes an ideal laxative for those who suffer from digestive disorders. It works great as an all-over body moisturizer or massage oil. Because of its relatively stable shelf life, it is great in body care products and facial blends. However, it needs to be mixed with another carrier oil that inhibits oxidation or an essential oil such as Benzoin. Sesame spreads easily all over the skin and leaves no greasy feeling.

Dilution: Use at 10% dilution with another carrier oil or carrier oil blend.

SHEA BUTTER is a thick, lustrous butter (not a carrier oil) with magnificent therapeutic properties. It leaves the skin feeling smooth and healthy and combats many skin conditions including dermatitis, eczema, burns, dry skin and more. Shea butter has a very rich consistency so you may want to warm and blend with other carrier oils for a thinner or liquid consistency if desired.

Dilution: Can be used at 100% or diluted at 25-25% with another carrier oil for blending purposes.

SUNFLOWER OIL has high amounts of Vitamins A, D and E as well as beneficial amounts of lecithin and unsaturated fatty acids. Its deeply nourishing benefits for the skin make it a favorite for recipes designed to treat dry, mature and damaged skin. It can be used for facial treatments and body massage as it offers satisfying softening and moisturizing properties. It also relieves the burn of sunburn. Sunflower oil is suitable for all skin types and frequently used for beauty and skin care products. It is considered an effective diuretic, helps with respiratory tract infections, especially if blended with sympathetic essential oils. This oil contains the highest level of vitamin E when compared to all the other vegetable oils. Vitamin E plays a role in normalizing blood pressure. Stores well under any condition but extreme heat and light will lessen the shelf life. It is not easily absorbed by the skin when applied and should be diluted with another carrier oil as a blend.

Dilution: Use at a 50% dilution with another carrier oil or carrier oil blend.

WALNUT OIL makes an excellent emollient with moisturizing properties for dry, aged, and irritated skin. This pale yellow oil works as a balancing agent for the nervous system. A study published in the Journal of the American College of Nutrition, examined walnuts and walnut oils, which contain polyunsaturated fats and their influence on blood pressure at rest and under stress and found it helps the body cope with stress by lowering resting blood pressure and blood pressure responses to stress. Previous studies showed that Omega-3 fatty acids—like the alpha linolenic acid found in walnuts and flax seeds—can reduce low density lipoproteins (LDL) and may reduce c-reactive protein and other markers of inflammation. Walnut oil can be used for massage and aromatherapy, however, it should be diluted with another carrier oil.

Dilution: Use at 10-25% dilution with another carrier oil or carrier oil blend.

WHEAT GERM OIL is high in Vitamin E, B1, B2, B3, B6, zinc, potassium, sulphur, phosphorus and other fatty acids that contain a natural antioxidant to help prevent rancidity. It can be added to other carrier oils to help prevent rancidity and lengthen their shelf life. Wheat Germ helps with its highly nourishing oil to promote the formation of new cells, improve circulation and repair sun damaged skin. It is also used to relieve the symptoms of dermatitis, psoriasis and eczema. Its consistency is extremely heavy and sticky which makes it not suitable to use as a carrier alone, but can be added to another carrier oil blend when mixing a massage oil. It is good for healing scar tissue, burns, wrinkles and stretch marks. Wheat Germ is known to internally strengthen the nervous system and helps remove the fatty plaque from arteries. It strengthens dry and split hair when massaged into the split ends for several minutes before washing.

Dilution: Use with other carrier oils at 5-10% dilution. Warning: May cause sensitization in some individuals.

DO NOT USE THESE

Mineral oil and petroleum jelly should never be used as a carrier oil in therapeutic blending. These are derivatives of petroleum production from gasoline and are not of natural botanical origins. Many commercially-based cosmetics and moisturizers contain mineral oil such as baby oil, because it is so inexpensive to manufacture. However, it clogs pores and prevents the skin from breathing naturally. In addition, it prevents toxins from escaping the body through perspiration and is believed to also prevent the body from properly absorbing vitamins and utilizing them, including essential oil absorption.

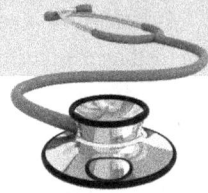

DILUTION RATE FOR YOUR
BLOOD PRESSURE BLENDS

When creating an essential oil blend for high blood pressure, you will need to take into consideration the percentage of dilution with a carrier oil. Be careful to dilute properly to make sure your blend is safe to use and doesn't waste your precious essential oil.

The following dilution rate chart shows you the percentage of pure therapeutic essential oil to use with the number of drops of carrier oil (vegetable oil) and will help you convert essential and carrier oil measurements. Use a measuring cup or spoon for carrier oils and pipettes for measuring your essential oils.

It is important to dilute your essential oil blend with a suitable carrier oil so that you can use it on the skin over a part of the body. There are several different carrier oils as mentioned earlier, such as Sweet Almond, cold-pressed Extra Virgin Olive, Flaxseed, Avocado, Grapeseed Extract, Jojoba, etc. You will want to select the best one for your condition and skin type. Carrier oils can be purchased from a natural health food store or grocer, but check labels to make sure the one you select is cold-pressed and is suitable for use on the skin.

In general, most essential oils should be diluted between 1%-5% with a carrier oil. For topical formulas, you will typically use 1-3% concentration of essential oils. This is 6-24 drops of essential oil per ounce of carrier. Therapeutic massage blends will contain between 1%-5% essential oils. However, each essential oil will have a different number of drops per milliliter, so to be more exact in your measuring, you will want to take this into consideration, too.

For instance, if you use two to three drops of pure essential oil, you will dilute by adding about a teaspoon of carrier oil. This should be cut in half for children and senior citizens.

SIMPLE EVERYDAY DILUTION CHART:

2-3 drops of Essential Oil per teaspoon of Carrier Oil

7-8 drops of Essential Oil per Tablespoon of Carrier Oil

15 drops of Essential Oil per ounce (30ml) of Carrier Oil

1 drop of essential oil = 1 tsp. of carrier oil for 1% dilution

2 drops of essential oil = 1 tsp. of carrier oil for 2% dilution

3 drops of essential oil = 1 tsp. of carrier oil for 3% dilution

4 drops of essential oil = 1 tsp. of carrier oil for 4% dilution

5 drops of essential oil = 1 tsp. of carrier oil for 5% dilution

Essential Oil	To	Carrier Oil
1 drop		¼ teaspoon
2-5 drops		1 teaspoon
4-10 drops		2 teaspoons
6-15 drops		1 Tablespoon
8-20 drops		4 teaspoons
12-30 drops		2 Tablespoons
Body Lotion		25

Essential Oil	To	Carrier Oil
Body Oil		50
Massage Oil		7-10
Shampoo		10
Conditioner		10
Chest Rub		15-25
Tissue		1-2
Mouthwash		2-3
Foot Bath/Spa		5
Bath		8-10
Shower		1-2

For general purposes, a blend is applied 6 times a day for acute conditions and 3-6 times a day for chronic complaints, or as needed.

MASSAGE OIL

When you use essential oils for a massage, you will definitely need to dilute with a carrier oil. Generally, two drops of therapeutic grade essential oil should be used per teaspoon of carrier oil (follow individual recipes when available). A full body massage takes about one to two ounces of carrier oil. Any natural carrier oil (except mineral oil) is fine to use when preparing a massage blend. As a general rule, add 10-12 drops of essential oil to 30ml of carrier oil. For children and elderly, use only 5-6 drops of essential oil to 30ml of carrier oil.

QUICK CONVERSIONS FOR DILUTION

Teaspoons to Drops
1/8 teaspoon = 12.5 drops = 1/48 ounce = 5/8 ml
1/4 teaspoon = 25 drops = 1/24 ounce = 1 1/4 ml
3/4 teaspoon = 75 drops = 1/8 ounce = 3.7 ml
1 teaspoon = 100 drops = 1/6 ounce = 5 ml

ML Conversion to Ounces (approximate drops)
1 ml = 20-24 drops
3 ml = .10 ounce (approximately 60-72 drops)

6 ml = .20 ounce (approximately 120-144 drops)

9 ml = .30 ounce (approximately 180-216 drops)

12 ml = .40 ounce (approximately 240-288 drops)

24 ml = .80 ounce (approximately 480-576 drops)

Quick Conversions

3 teaspoons (tsp.) = 1 Tablespoon (Tbsp.)

2 Tablespoons (Tbsp.) = 1 ounce (oz.)

6 teaspoons (tsp.) = 1 ounce (oz.)

10 milliliter (ml) = 1/3 ounce (oz.)

15 milliliter (ml) = 1/2 ounce (oz.)

30 milliliter (ml) = 1 ounce (oz.)

10 milliliter (ml) = approximately 300 drops

1% Dilution Rate (approximate)

1 ounce carrier oil (2 Tablespoons) + 6 drops essential oil

2 ounces carrier oil (1/4 cup) + 12 drops essential oil

3 ounces carrier oil (1/3 cup) + 18 drops essential oil

4 ounces carrier oil (1/2 cup) + 24 drops (or 1 ml) essential oil

8 ounces carrier oil (1 cup) + 48 drops (or 2 ml) essential oil

2% Dilution Rate (approximate)

1 ounce carrier oil (2 Tablespoons) + 12 drops essential oil

2 ounces carrier oil (1/4 cup) + 24 drops (or 1 ml) essential oil

3 ounces carrier oil (1/3 cup) + 36 drops (or 1½ ml) essential oil

4 ounces carrier oil (1/2 cup) + 48 drops (or 2 ml) essential oil

8 ounces carrier oil (1 cup) + 96 drops (or 4 ml) essential oil

3% Dilution Rate (approximate)

1 ounce carrier oil (2 Tablespoons) + 18 drops essential oil

2 ounces carrier oil (1/4 cup) + 36 drops (or 1½ ml) essential oil

3 ounces carrier oil (1/3 cup) + 44 drops (or 2 ml) essential oil

4 ounces carrier oil (1/2 cup) + 72 drops (or 3 ml) essential oil

8 ounces carrier oil (1 cup) + 144 drops (or 6 ml) essential oil

5% Dilution Rate (approximate)

1 ounce carrier oil (2 Tablespoons) + 1.5 ml essential oil

2 ounces carrier oil (1/4 cup) + 3 ml essential oil

3 ounces carrier oil (1/3 cup) + 4.5 ml essential oil

4 ounces carrier oil (1/2 cup) + 6 ml essential oil

8 ounces carrier oil (1 cup) + 9 ml essential oil

10% Dilution Rate (approximate)

1 ounce carrier oil (2 Tablespoons) + 3 ml essential oil

2 ounces carrier oil (1/4 cup) + 6 ml essential oil

3 ounces carrier oil (1/3 cup) + 9 ml essential oil

4 ounces carrier oil (1/2 cup) + 12 ml essential oil

8 ounces carrier oil (1 cup) + 24 ml essential oil

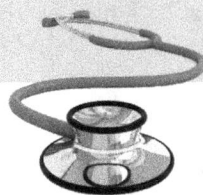

EQUIPMENT USED WHEN CREATING BLENDS FOR
HIGH BLOOD PRESSURE

Before getting started, you will want to gather the supplies you will need such as bottles, droppers, and containers. Below is a list of the basic tools you will need to have on hand:

Glass Bottles, preferably dark, in 5ml, 10ml, and 15ml sizes with orifice reducers (plastic dropper) can be used to make topical essential oil blends.

Plastic Bottles with a pump, squirt, or screw off top are suitable for liquid soaps, shower gels, shampoos, lotions, and conditioners. You can find these in 2-ounce, 4-ounce, and 8-ounce sizes.

Plastic or Glass Spray Bottles are great to have on hand when making room sprays, facial spritzers or cleaning solutions. You will find these in 1-ounce, 2-ounce, 4-ounce, 8-ounce and 16-ounce sizes.

Small Glass or Plastic Tubs are perfect for bath salts, facial creams, salves, scrubs or other bath blends. These come in a variety of shapes and sizes from 2-ounce to 8-ounce.

Pocket Diffusers are perfect as "personal inhalers" to carry in a pocket or purse with your favorite blend. They come with a cotton wick that saturates the essential oil inside the chamber. These are terrific for taking to work or school!

Plastic Transfer Pipettes come in different sizes and lengths for easy and precise drop measuring. They are ideal for filling small vials and for measure dropping small amounts of oils. Use these when you want to transfer oil from a large bottle into smaller bottles. They are for one time use and should be thrown away to avoid cross-contamination.

Clear Mini Atomizers are perfect for trips. You can use these to make and share with friends and family (1ml or 2ml sizes work best).

You will need waterproof labels for your bottles and you will want them in all shapes and sizes. Visit Online Labels for a wide variety of sizes at http://www.onlinelabels.com/.

Items such as bottles and pipettes are available online at SKS Bottle & Packaging and Rachel's Supply.

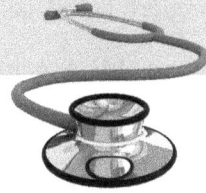

BIBLIOGRAPHY

Aourell M, Skoog M, Carleson J 2005 Effects of Swedish massage on blood pressure. Complementary Therapies in Clinical Practice 11:242-246

Aviram M, Dornfeld L, Rosenblat M, et al. Pomegranate juice consumption reduces oxidative stress, atherogenic modifications to LDL, and platelet aggregation:studies in humans and in atherosclerotic apolipoprotein E-deficient mice. Am J Clin Nutr 2000;71(5):1062-76. Aviram M, Dornfeld L. Pomegranate juice consumption inhibits serum angiotensin converting enzyme activity and reduces systolic blood pressure. Atherosclerosis 2001;158(1):195-8.

Aydin Y, Kutlay O, Ari S et al 2007 Hypotensive effects of carvacrol on the blood pressure of normotensive rats.

Battaglia, Salvatore, 2007, *The Complete Guide to Aromatherapy*, The Healing Arts Press

Battaglia Salvatore, 1997, *The Complete Guide to Aromatherapy*. The Perfect Potion, Virginia, Queensland

Caujolle F, Franck C 1945a Pharmacodynamic actions of clary sage and condiment sage. Comptes Rendues Société Biologique 139:1109-1110

Clarke, Sue, 2008, *Essential Chemistry for Aromatherapy*, Elsevier Limited

Chobanian AV, et al. and the National High Blood Pressure Education Program Coordinating Committee. The seventh report of the Joint National Committee on Prevention, Detection, Evaluation, and Treatment of High Blood Pressure: The JNC 7 report. JAMA. 2003;298:2560-2572.

Christensen BV, Lynch HJ 1937 A comparative study of the pharmacological actions of natural and synthetic camphor.

Coombs HC, Pike FH 1931 Respiratory and cardiovascular changes in the cat during convulsions of experimental origin. The American Journal of Physiology 97:92-106

Davis P 1999 *Aromatherapy an A-Z*. CW Daniel, Saffron Walden

Dawson AN, Walser B, Jafarzadeh M et al 2004 Topical analgesics and blood pressure during static contraction in humans. Medicine & Science in Sports & Exercise 36:632-638

Dayawansa S, Umeno K, Takakura H et al 2003 Autonomic responses during inhalation of natural fragrance of cedrol in humans. Autonomic Neuroscience 108:79-86

Franchomme P, Pénöel D 1990 *L'aromathérapie exactement*. Jollois, Limoges

Futami T 1984 [Actions and mechanisms of counterirritants on the muscular circulation]. Nippon Yakurigaku Zasshi 83:219-226

Gattefosse, M. (1992) *Gattefosse's aromatherapy* (translated by Tisserand, R). Saffron Walden, C W Daniel.

Gaziano JM, Ridker PM, Libby P. Primary and secondary prevention of coronary heart disease. In: Bonow RO, Mann DL, Zipes DP, Libby P, eds. *Braunwald's Heart Disease: A Textbook of Cardiovascular Medicine*. 9th ed. Saunders; 2011:chap 49.

Goldstein LB, Bushnell CD, Adams RJ, et al. Guidelines for the primary prevention of stroke: a guideline for healthcare professionals from the American Heart Association/American Stroke Association. Stroke. 2011 Feb;42:517-84.

Greenberg B and Kahn AM. Clinical assessment of heart failure. In: Bonow RO, Mann DL, Zipes DP, Libby P, eds. *Braunwald's Heart Disease: A Textbook of Cardiovascular Medicine*. 9th ed. Saunders; 2011:chap 26.

Haze S, Sakai K, Gozu Y 2002 Effects of fragrance inhalation on sympathetic activity in normal adults. Japanese

Hills JM, Aaronson PI 1991 The mechanism of action of peppermint oil on gastrointestinal smooth muscle.

Jessup M, Abraham WT, Casey DE, Feldman AM, Francis GS, Ganiats TG, et al. 2009 focused update: ACCF/AHA Guidelines for the Diagnosis and Management of Heart Failure in Adults: a report of the American College of Cardiology Foundation/American Heart Association Task Force on Practice Guidelines: developed in collaboration with the International Society for Heart and Lung Transplantation. Circulation. 2009 Apr 14;119(14):1977-2016. Epub 2009 Mar 26.

Joint National Committee on Detection, Evaluation, and Treatment of Blood Pressure. The seventh report of the joint national committee on detection, evaluation, and treatment of blood pressure. NIH Publication No. 03-5233, May, 2003.

Journal of the American Pharmaceutical Association 26:786-96

Journal of Pharmacology 90:247-253Heuberger E, Hongratanaworakit T, Bohm C et al 2001 Effects of chiral fragrances on human autonomic nervous system parameters and self-evaluation. Chemical Senses 26:281-292

Kaplan NM. Systemic hypertension: Treatment. In: Bonow RO, Mann DL, Zipes DP, Libby P, eds. *Braunwald's Heart Disease: A Textbook of Cardiovascular Medicine.* 9th ed. Philadelphia, Pa: Saunders Elsevier; 2011:chap 46.

Kulieva ZT 1980 [Analgesic, hypotensive and cardiotonic action of the essential oil of thyme growing in Azerbaijan].

Lahlou S, Figueiredo AF, Magalhães PJ et al 2002 Cardiovascular effects of 1,8-cineole, a terpenoid oxide present in many plant essential oils, in normotensive rats. Canadian Journal of Physiology & Pharmacology 80:1125-1131

Lahlou S, Magalhaes PJ, de Siqueira RJ et al 2005 Cardiovascular effects of the essential oil of Aniba canelilla bark in normotensive rats. Journal of Cardiovascular Pharmacology 46:412-421

Magyar J, Szentandrassy N, Banyasz T et al 2004 Effects of terpenoid phenol derivatives on calcium current in canine and human ventricular cardiomyocytes. European Journal of Pharmacology 487:29-36

Mant J, Al-Mohammad A, Swain S, Laramée P; Guideline Development Group. Management of chronic heart failure in adults: synopsis of the National Institute For Health and Clinical Excellence guideline. Ann Intern Med. 2011 Aug16;155(4):252-9.

McNamara ME, Burnham DC, Smith C et al 2003 The effects of back massage before diagnostic cardiac catheterization. Alternative Therapies in Health & Medicine 9:50-57

Mercola.com, Dr. Paul J. Rosch interview with Dr. John Laragh, *Why the Treatment of Hypertension Has Become Such a Deplorable Fiasco*, Part I, (Accessed 9/2/08)

Mojay, Gabriel, 1997, *Aromatherapy for Healing the Spirit*, Gaia Books Ltd

Northover BJ, Verghese J 1962 The pharmacology of certain terpene alcohols and oxides. Journal of Scientific & Industrial Research 21C:342-345

Peng SM, Koo M, Yu ZR., 2009 Jan, Effects of music and essential oil inhalation on cardiac autonomic balance in healthy individuals, J Altern Complement Med, 15(1):53-7

Pitman V 2004 *Aromatherapy: A Practical Approach*. Nelson Thornes, Cheltenham

Ragan BG, Nelson AJ, Foreman JH et al 2004 Effects of a menthol-based analgesic balm on pressor responses evoked from muscle afferents in cats. American Journal of Veterinary Research 65:1204-1210

Riegel B, Moser DK, Anker SD, et al; American Heart Association Council on Cardiovascular Nursing; American Heart Association Council on Clinical Cardiology; American Heart Association Council on Nutrition, Physical Activity, and Metabolism; American Heart Association Interdisciplinary Council on Quality of Care and Outcomes Research. State of the science: promoting self-care in persons with heart failure: a scientific statement from the American Heart Association. Circulation. 2009 Sep 22;120(12):1141-63.

Rose, J. (1994): *Guide to Essential Oils*. San Francisco, CA. Jeanne Rose Aromatherapy.

Seo JY., 2009 Jun, The effects of aromatherapy on stress and stress responses in adolescents, J Korean Acad Nursing, 39(3):357-65.

Tiran, D. (1996): *Aromatherapy in Midwifery Practice*. London, Bailliere Tindall.

Tisserand, R. (1994, 1977): *The Art of Aromatherapy*. Saffron Walden, The C W Daniel Co Ltd.

Tisserand, R. and Balacs, T. (1995): *Essential Oil Safety*. London, Churchill Livingstone.

Todorov S, Philianos S, Petkov V et al 1984 Experimental pharmacological study of three species from genus Salvia.

Totilo, Rebecca Park, 2013, *Therapeutic Blending With Essential Oil*, Rebecca at the Well Foundation

Touvay C, Vilain B, Carre C et al 1995 Effect of limonene and sobrerol on monocrotaline-induced lung alterations and pulmonary hypertension. International Archives of Allergy & Immunology 107:272-274Valnet J 1964 Aromathérapie. Librairie Maloine, Paris (English translation: Valnet J 1990 The practice of aromatherapy. CW Daniel, Saffron Walden)

Victor RG. Arterial hypertension. In: Goldman L, Schafer AI, eds. Cecil Medicine. 24th ed. Saunders; 2011:chap 67, 220.

Victor RG. Systemic hypertension: Mechanisms and diagnosis. In: Bonow RO, Mann DL, Zipes DP, Libby P, eds. *Braunwald's Heart Disease: A Textbook of Cardiovascular Medicine*. 9th ed. Philadelphia, Pa: Saunders Elsevier; 2011:chap 45.

OTHER BOOKS BY REBECCA PARK TOTILO

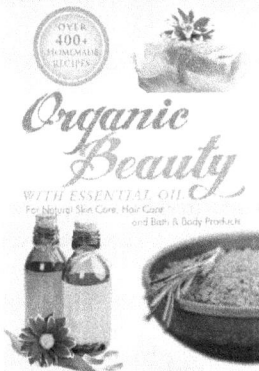

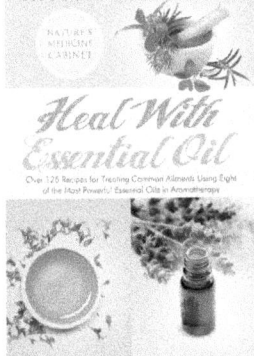

Organic Beauty With Essential Oil: Over 400+ Homemade Recipes for Natural Skin Care, Hair Care and Bath & Body Products

Sweep aside all those harmful chemically-based cosmetics and make your own organic bath and body products at home with the magic of potent essential oils! In this book, you'll find a luxurious array of over 400 Eco-friendly recipes that call for breathtaking fragrances and soothing, rich organic ingredients satisfying you head to toe. Included you'll find helpful can have the confidence knowing which essential oil to use and how much when creating your own body scrub, lip butter, or lotion bar! Discover how easy it is to make bath treats like fragrant shower gels, dreamy bubble baths, luscious creams and lotions, deep cleansing masks and facials for literally pennies using only a few essential oils and ingredients from your own kitchen with Organic Beauty with Essential Oil.

Heal With Essential Oil: Nature's Medicine Cabinet

Using essential oils drawn from nature's own medicine cabinet of flowers, trees, seeds and roots, man can tap into God's healing power to heal oneself from almost any pain. Find relief from many conditions and rejuvenate the body. With over 125 recipes, this practical guide will walk you through in the most easy-to-understand form how to treat common ailments with your essential oils for everyday living. Filled with practical advice on therapeutic blending of oils and safety, a directory of the most effective oils for common ailments and easy to follow remedies chart , and prescriptive blends for aches, pains and sicknesses.

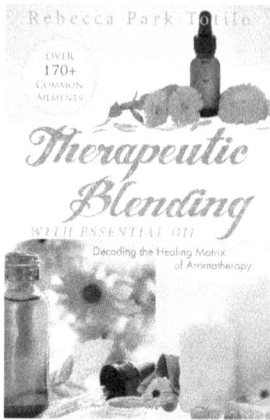

Therapeutic Blending With Essential Oil: Decoding the Healing Matrix of Aromatherapy

Therapeutic Blending With Essential Oil unlocks the healing power of essential oils and guides you through the intricate matrix of aromatherapy, with a compilation of over 170 common ailments.

Discover how to properly formulate a blend for any physical or emotional symptom with easy to follow customizable recipes. Now, you can make your own personalized massage oils, hand and body lotions, bath gels, compresses, salve ointments, smelling salts, nasal inhalers and more. This exhaustive guide takes all the guesswork out of blending essential oils from how many drops to include in a blend, to working with and measuring thick oils, to how often to apply it for acute or chronic conditions. It also shows you how to create a single blend for multiple conditions. Even if you run out of oil for a favorite recipe, this book shows you how to substitute it with another oil.

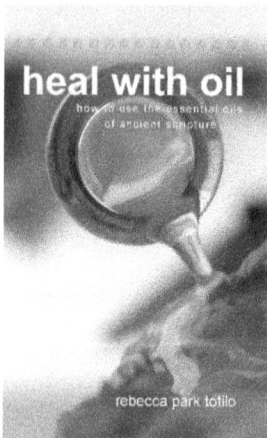

Heal With Oil: How to Use the Essential Oils of Ancient Scripture

God has provided a natural remedy to our Healthcare crisis - essential oils extracted from plants and trees. In this practical guide, Rebecca instructs believers on how to use the twelve healing oils mentioned in Holy Scriptures for healing and restoration of the body. Learn about the hidden treasures of the Levitical Priests and what the pharmaceutical companies don't want you to know. Book includes practical advice on blending oils and safety, a directory of properties for twelve oils from the Bible and special blends for the bath and personal care. Tons of recipes for beauty, health and emotional well-being.

Heal With Essential Oil
nature's medicine cabinet

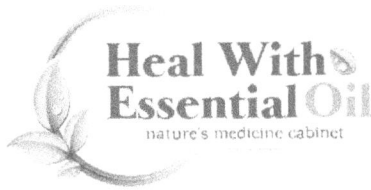

For other books, DVDs, and essential oils products, please visit our website:

http://HealWithEssentialOil.com

For e-mail correspondence, please write:

info@healwithessentialoil.com

For snail mail correspondence:

Heal With Essential Oil
P.O. Box 60044
St. Petersburg, FL 33784

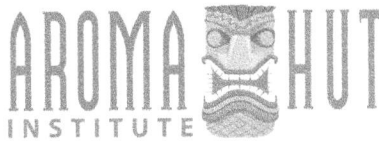

AROMA HUT
INSTITUTE

For more information about our aromatherapy certification programs, please visit our website:

http://AromaHut.org

For e-mail correspondence, please write:

info@AromaHut.org

Please visit our training facilities and retail shop at:

Aroma Hut Institute
4930 Park Blvd. N.
Suite 9
Pinellas Park, FL 33781

www.ingramcontent.com/pod-product-compliance
Lightning Source LLC
Chambersburg PA
CBHW071137280326
41935CB00010B/1267